PEDIATRIC EYE DISEASE
COLOR ATLAS AND SYNOPSIS

PEDIATRIC EYE DISEASE

COLOR ATLAS AND SYNOPSIS

Richard W. Hertle, M.D., F.A.C.S., F.A.A.O.

Pediatric Ophthalmology, Strabismus, and Eye Movement Disorders
The Laboratory of Sensorimotor Research
The National Eye Institute, The National Institutes of Health
Consultant, The Department of Ophthalmology
The National Naval Medical Center
Bethesda, Maryland
The Walter Reed Army Medical Center
Washington, D.C.

David B. Schaffer, M.D.

Former Professor of Ophthalmology
Department of Ophthalmology
The University of Pennsylvania School of Medicine
Chief of Pediatric Ophthalmology
The Children's Hospital of Philadelphia
Philadelphia, Pennsylvania

Jill A. Foster, M.D., F.A.C.S.

Ophthalmic Plastic and Reconstructive Surgery
Clinical Assistant Professor
Department of Ophthalmology
Grant Eye and Ear Hospital
Ohio State University
Columbus, Ohio

McGRAW-HILL
MEDICAL PUBLISHING DIVISION

New York   Chicago   San Francisco   Lisbon   London   Madrid   Mexico City   Milan   New Delhi
San Juan   Seoul   Singapore   Sydney   Toronto

McGraw-Hill

A Division of The **McGraw·Hill** *Companies*

PEDIATRIC EYE DISEASE
COLOR ATLAS AND SYNOPSIS

1234567890 IMP IMP 0987654321

ISBN 0-07-136509-5

This book was set in Times Roman by North Market Street Graphics.
The editors were Darlene Barela Cooke, Susan R. Noujaim, and Muza Navrozov.
The production supervisor was Catherine H. Saggese.
The designer was Marsha Cohen/Parallelogram.
The index was done by Alexandra Nickerson.
Imago was printer and binder.

This book is printed on recycled, acid-free paper.

Library of Congress Cataloging-in-Publication Data

Pediatric eye disease: color atlas and synopsis / editors, Richard W. Hertle,
David B. Schaffer, Jill A. Foster.
      p. cm.
    Includes bibliographical references and index.
    ISBN 0-07-136509-5 (alk. paper)
    1. Pediatric ophthalmology—Atlases.   I. Hertle, Richard W.
II. Schaffer, David B.   III. Foster, Jill A.
   [DNLM: 1. Eye Diseases—Child—Atlases.   WW 17 C641 2002]
RE48.2.C5 C55 2001
618.92'0977—dc21   2001030012

To my wife Gloriann

Only her talent and energies as a loving mother, teacher, and child-care professional surpass her daily support of my personal and professional passions. She is an inspiration to me and a role model for any young woman who desires to overcome the complicated and diverse demands required by our times.

RWH

CONTENTS

PART I
NEONATAL EYE DISEASE / 1

PART II
OPHTHALMIC DISEASE IN INFANTS / 57

P A R T   I I I
OPHTHALMIC DISEASE IN TODDLERS / 117

P A R T   I V
OPHTHALMIC DISEASE IN SCHOOL-AGE CHILDREN / 179

James J. Augsberger, M.D. [17]
Professor and Chairman
Department of Ophthalmology
University of Cincinnati College of Medicine
Cincinnati, Ohio

John M. Avallone, M.D. [7, 13]
CAPT, MC, USN Ophthalmology
Director, Pediatric Ophthalmology Service
National Naval Medical Center
Associate Professor, Uniformed Services University
    of the Health Sciences
Bethesda, Maryland

Gordon Byrnes, M.D. [23]
CAPT, MC, USN Ophthalmology
Vitreoretinal Surgery Service
National Naval Medical Center
Associate Professor, Uniformed Services University
    of the Health Sciences
Bethesda, Maryland

Edward W. Cheeseman, M.D. [14]
CAPT, MC, USN Ophthalmology
Pediatric Ophthalmology Staff
National Naval Medical Center
Associate Professor
Uniformed Services University of the Health Sciences
Bethesda, Maryland

Cindy W. Christian, M.D. [11]
Assistant Professor of Pediatrics
University of Pennsylvania School of Medicine
Director, Child Abuse Services
The Children's Hospital of Philadelphia
Philadelphia, Pennsylvania

Edmond J. FitzGibbon, M.D. [10]
Neuroophthalmology Service
The Laboratory of Sensorimotor Research
The National Eye Institute
The National Institutes of Health
Bethesda, Maryland

Jill A. Foster, M.D., F.A.C.S. [5, 8, 15, 22]
Ophthalmic Plastic and Reconstructive Surgery
Clinical Assistant Professor
Department of Ophthalmology
Grant Eye and Ear Hospital
Ohio State University
Columbus, Ohio

David B. Granet, M.D., F.A.C.S., F.A.A.P., F.A.A.O. [20]
Director, Pediatric Ophthalmology &
    Strabismus Services
UCSD/Ratner Children's Eye Center
Associate Professor
Departments of Ophthalmology and Pediatrics
University of California
San Diego, California

Barrett G. Haik, M.D., F.A.C.S. [16]
Hamilton Professor and Chair
Department of Ophthalmology
University of Tennessee Health Science Center
Department of Surgery
St. Jude Children's Research Hospital
Memphis, Tennessee

Richard W. Hertle, M.D., F.A.C.S., F.A.A.O. [1, 4, 8]
Pediatric Ophthalmology, Strabismus, and
    Eye Movement Disorders
The Laboratory of Sensorimotor Research
The National Eye Institute
The National Institutes of Health
Consultant, The Departments of Ophthalmology
The National Naval Medical Center
Bethesda, Maryland
The Walter Reed Army Medical Center
Washington, D.C.

*Numbers in brackets following the contributor's name refer to chapters written or cowritten by the contributor.

David E. Holck, M.D. [15]

Director, Oculoplastic, Orbital &
   Ocular Oncology Service
Department of Ophthalmology
Wilford Hall Medical Center
San Antonio, Texas

Scot Lance, M.D., F.A.C.S. [12]

Clinical Instructor, Department of Ophthalmology
Oculoplastic Service
The University of South Florida
Sarasota, Florida

Wendy G. Lane, M.D., M.P.H. [11]

University of Pennsylvania School of Medicine
Child Abuse Services
The Children's Hospital of Philadelphia
Philadelphia, Pennsylvania

William Madigan III, M.D., COL [3]

Director, Pediatric Ophthalmology
Walter Reed Army Medical Center
Washington, D.C.

Albert M. Maguire, M.D. [9]

Associate Professor, Department of Ophthalmology
The University of Pennsylvania School of Medicine
Chief, Retina Service, The Scheie Eye Institute
Consultant, Department of Ophthalmology
The Children's Hospital of Philadelphia
Philadelphia, Pennsylvania

Mitra Maybodi, M.D. [19]

Fellow, Pediatric Ophthalmology, Strabismus,
   and Eye Movement Disorders
The Laboratory of Sensorimotor Research
The National Eye Institute
The National Institutes of Health
Bethesda, Maryland

Robert B. Nussenblatt, M.D. [18]

Head, The Laboratory of Immunology
Scientific Director, Intramural Program
The National Eye Institute
The National Institutes of Health
Bethesda, Maryland

John Ort, Certified Optician [24]

Aristocraft Opticians
Hauppauge, New York

Julian D. Perry, M.D. [22]

Head, Department of Ophthalmic Plastic
   and Reconstructive Surgery
Division of Ophthalmology
The Cleveland Clinic Foundation
Cleveland, Ohio

David F. Plotsky, M.D. [21]

Director of Pediatric Ophthalmology
   and Strabismus Service
Washington National Eye Center
Washington, D.C.

Charles B. Pratt, M.D. [16]

Department of Oncology
St. Jude Children's Research Hospital
Memphis, Tennessee

Chaundra Roy, M.D. [18]

Fellow, The Laboratory of Immunology
The National Eye Institute
The National Institutes of Health
Bethesda, Maryland

David B. Schaffer, M.D. [2, 6, 14]

Former Professor of Ophthalmology
The Department of Ophthalmology
The University of Pennsylvania School of Medicine
Chief of Pediatric Ophthalmology
The Children's Hospital of Philadelphia
Philadelphia, Pennsylvania

John T. Tong, M.D. [5]

Division of Ophthalmic Plastic
   and Reconstructive Surgery
Jules Stein Eye Institute
University of California, Los Angeles
Los Angeles, California

Matthew W. Wilson, M.D. [16]

Assistant Professor,
Department of Ophthalmology
University of Tennessee Health Science Center
Department of Surgery
St. Jude Children's Research Hospital
Memphis, Tennessee

Terri L. Young, M.D. [6]

Associate Professor of Medicine
The University of Pennsylvania School of Medicine
Staff, Division of Ophthalmology
The Children's Hospital of Philadelphia
Philadelphia, Pennsylvania

The idea for this atlas originated with the generous gift from David B. Schaffer, M.D., of his 30-year collection of clinical photographs to me upon his retirement. His attention to detail in the collection, categorization, and preservation of this material inspired me to keep this material from collecting dust for the next 30 years. Using these photographs only for selected lectures was not doing them justice. I felt that this collection could be better used in publication form for a wider audience. With the aid and support of Ms. Darlene Cooke of McGraw-Hill, the proposal for this atlas became more purposeful and began to take on life. As the idea for this atlas took shape, the other editors and I decided that participation of other eye care professionals would provide a diversity of opinion and experience that truly represents the needs and eye diseases of infants and children. The added benefit of this participation was the consolidation of their figures, photos, and thoughts with those of the editors, thus providing a more complete compilation of materials.

There are multiple purposes to this atlas. Our first goal was to provide a varied, visual representation of the more common eye diseases that present in infancy and childhood. We understand that no book can show the hundreds of diseases presenting in hundreds of ways; however, with the support of the publisher we have been able to publish about 450 photographs (about 400 in color), which illustrate the variation in appearance of many childhood eye diseases. We organized the text so as to highlight definitions of terms, differential diagnosis, workup, and major treatment options. We do not wish to replace the many excellent texts covering the diagnosis and treatment of pediatric eye diseases and strabismus, but we do wish to photographically enhance these texts. We have created this atlas to serve as a reference material to be used by the many people involved with infants and children— pediatric physicians and nurses, family care personnel, child day care centers, emergency rooms, schools, optometrists, opticians, ophthalmologists, and those who come in daily contact with infants and children.

We have divided this atlas into five major parts, which reflect, as much as possible, those diseases that more commonly present in neonates (Part I), infants (Part II), toddlers (Part III), school-age children (Part IV), and other common childhood eye problems (Part V). We understand that there may be considerable overlap in the age of presentation of these eye diseases, but we felt that this format would allow the busy professional examining a child the most direct route of photographic reference. Neonatal eye diseases include ophthalmia neonatorum, TORCH syndromes, cataracts, glaucoma, retinopathy of prematurity, and congenital anomalies of the lids and orbit. Infantile diseases include strabismus, genetic and craniofacial syndromes, vitreoretinal diseases, optic nerve anomalies, nonaccidental trauma, and nasolacrimal duct obstruction. Problems in toddlers include amblyopia and strabismus, infections and inflammations, ptosis, and orbital and eye tumors. Diseases in school-age children include uveitis, nystagmus and anomalous head positions, vision development, testing and visual screening, and refractive errors. Other common problems include accidental trauma and spectacles in infants and children.

We feel that the specific addition of chapters on nonaccidental trauma (abuse and neglect) vision testing and screening and spectacles in children provide unique additions to an atlas of this type. The illustration of these common eye conditions and childhood needs should provide any professional caring for infants and children special insights. These may be particularly useful for the non-eye care professional in that they emphasize salient clinical characteristics and testing procedures encountered in common childhood eye situations.

We understand that the rapidly changing technology, transfer of information, and almost daily acquisition of new knowledge create challenges to the medical educator. This is true whether one is educating health care professionals, students, or patients and families. This pressure to provide "up-to-date" information is a prevalent part of our times and drastically complicates the publishing process. This atlas is unique and timely in that, while our understanding and treatments of eye diseases in infants and children are constantly changing, the appearance of these diseases is almost timeless. We believe that this timeless appearance of eye diseases in infants and children will be the foundation of this atlas as a long-standing reference for those who have the fortune and pleasure of working with children.

This section allows a contemplative assessment of where one is how one got there. For me this is not a recitation of places but of people. I would like to thank all the families that trusted us with their most precious gift, their children. If not for these patients, this book would not have been possible. I would next like to thank all the contributing authors, who interrupted their busy lives and provided a unique dedication to their authorship task. Throughout my personal life and professional career, there have been people who have believed in my ideals, supported my plans, encouraged my passion for ophthalmology and guided my sometimes wayward energies. All these people are fundamentally responsible for the completion of this book. My parents Ann and Richard and brothers and sister, Steve, Jim, and Sue provided me with the values of a strong work ethic, loyalty to family and friends and honesty at work and home. My stepchildren Jessica and Jamie have given me the privilege of being a parent. The late Malio Cascardo was there during my tumultuous teen years and provided a professional and personal sanctuary. As an undergraduate student in Columbus, Ohio, Robert Hagman II of Ohio State Optical Co. and Gary L. Rogers, M.D., each gave me opportunities to shape my professional work in eye care and medical research. During my medical training in Northeastern Ohio, the late Hayes Davis, M.D., was a powerful mentor to me, as he was for many students, and Scot E. Lance, M.D., became my friend for life. Mohammed Ashrafzadeh, M.D., practically "gave" me all his surgical skills and was a beacon of light and calm during the storm of residency in Boston. Louis F. Dell'Osso, Ph.D., has been, and remains, a mentor and friend. David B. Schaffer, M.D., Glen A. Gole, M.D., James A. Katowitz, M.D., and Arthur J. Jampolsky, M.D., took the time to show me the skills needed to become an expert in pediatric ophthalmology and strabismus. In recent years Marshall M. Parks, M.D., has embraced me and provided community support for my pediatric ophthalmology clinical research service at the National Eye Institute. Last, I would like to thank the Residents in Ophthalmology at The University of Pennsylvania, The Walter Reed Army Medical Center, and The Washington Hospital Center as well as those Fellows in pediatric ophthalmology who have worked with me over the years. Their constant questioning, desire for knowledge and dedication to the care of children have forced me to stay sharp. Those previous Fellows include David B. Granet, M.D., Joseph A. Napolitano, M.D., Sule Ziylan, M.D., Gary D. Markowitz, M.D., Martin C. Wilson, M.D., Yvette M. Jockin, M.D., Sepidah L. Rousta, M.D., Darron A. Bacal, M.D., Mitra Maybodi, M.D., and Michael Schaffer, M.D.

Richard W. Hertle

PART I

NEONATAL EYE DISEASE

OPHTHALMIA NEONATORUM

RICHARD W. HERTLE

DEFINITION OF TERMS

Ophthalmia neonatorum (ON) is an inflammatory disease of the ocular surface occurring in the first 28 to 30 days of life. It is usually caused by *Neisseria gonorrhoeae* infection. In the 1880s Crede's use of silver nitrate as prophylaxis against ON was a remarkable medical and public health achievement, because it decreased the incidence of newborn conjunctivitis from 10% to 0.3%. The Centers for Disease Control (CDC) reported 900,000 cases of ON in 1986.

DIFFERENTIAL DIAGNOSIS

The most common causes reflect the infectious nature of this condition and include the following:

1. *N. gonorrhoeae*
2. *Chlamydia trachomatis* (about 20% of neonates will suffer from associated systemic involvement)
3. Bacterial conjunctivitis (staphylococci, streptococci, *Haemophilus* species, coliform groups)
4. Viral conjunctivitis and keratitis (most commonly herpes simplex types I and II).
5. Chemical conjunctivitis (silver nitrate)
6. Ocular trauma
7. Congenital glaucoma
8. Congenital lacrimal system obstruction

WORKUP

1. Parental history of sexually transmitted diseases
2. Complete ophthalmic examination
3. Cytologic analysis of ocular discharge (Gram stain, Giemsa stain, Wright stain)
4. Immunofluorescent antibodies (*Chlamydia* infection)
5. Fluorescein-conjugated antibodies of McCoy cell cultures (*Chlamydia* infection)
6. Cultures (aerobic, anaerobic, and viral infections)
7. Immunocytochemical diagnosis (viral infections)

TREATMENT (See Table 1-1 on page 4)

1. Topical and systemic antibiotics (various combinations of penicillins, erythromycin, cephalosporins, and antiherpetic agents)
2. Irrigation of the ocular surface
3. Treatment of parents and their sexual contacts

CONCLUSIONS

The impact of 100 years of prophylaxis in preventing and decreasing the prevalence of blinding disease from ON in neonates must not lead to complacency. Until predisposing conditions are eliminated, this remains a potentially significant medical problem.

SUGGESTED TREATMENT APPROACH FOR NEONATAL CONJUNCTIVITIS*

Diagnosis (by History and Physical and Laboratory Evaluations)	Treatment
1. *Chlamydia trachomatis* (see Figs. 1-5–1-7)	Ocular—Erythromycin ointment O U qid × 2 weeks Systemic—Erythromycin 30–40 mg/kg/d po × 2 weeks
2. *Neisseria gonorrhoeae* (see Figs. 1-1–1-4)	Ocular—Erythromycin ointment O U qid × 2 weeks and topical ocular irrigation Systemic—Aqueous penicillin G, 100,000 U/kg/d I V qid × 7 days or ceftriaxone, 28–50 mg/kg/d I V q8–12 h × 7 days
3. Herpes simplex (see Figs. 1-8–1-10)	Ocular—Trifluorothymidine (Viroptic) 9 times qd × 14 days Systemic—+/– Acyclovir (Zovirax) IV solution
4. Other viral or epidemic (see Figs. 1-12–1-13)	Ocular—Cool compresses, +/– erythromycin ointment or polymyxin B solution qid × 7 days Systemic—Supportive treatment
5. Chemical (see Fig. 1-11)	Ocular—Self-limited, observation only

*If a corneal ulcer is suspected or diagnosed (topical fluoroscein staining of the cornea is positive), prompt ophthalmic referral is indicated.

Key: +/–, means no problem using or not using —usually used when there are signs of secondary bacterial involvement.

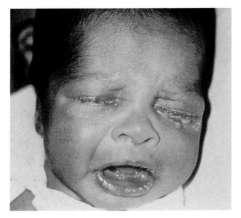

Figure 1-1

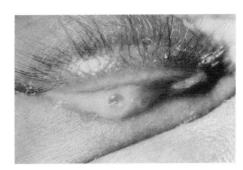

Figure 1-2

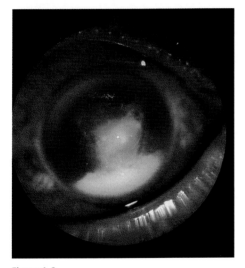

Figure 1-3

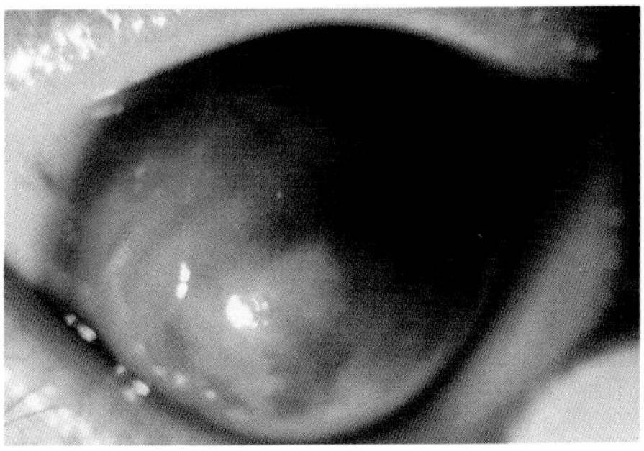

Figure 1-4

Figures 1-1 to 1-4 *These figures depict the spectrum of involvement of the conjunctiva, corneal surface, and eye in* Neisseria gonorrhoeae *infection. Figures 1-1 and 1-2 show the copious mucopurulent conjunctival discharge that is a clinical characteristic of this infection. Figure 1-3 shows progression of the infection to include the cornea, producing ulcerative keratitis and a hypopyon ("pus" in the anterior chamber). Figure 1-4 shows end-stage panophthalmitis with infection of the intraocular contents with secondary corneal thinning and ectasia with the possibility of prolapse of intraocular contents through the cornea.*

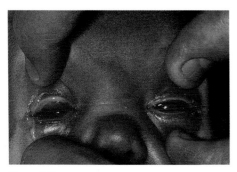

Figure 1-5

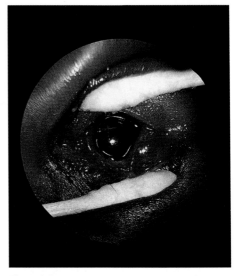

Figure 1-6

Figures 1-5 to 1-7 *These figures depict the spectrum of involvement of the conjunctival surface. Figure 1-5 shows bilateral lid edema, erythema, and watery discharge more characteristic of chlamydial conjunctivitis. Figures 1-6 and 1-7 show the intense, diffuse palpebral hyperemia and occasional membrane formation (arrow in Fig. 1-7) with this infection.*

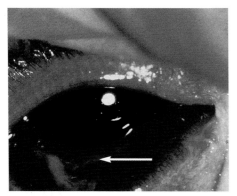

Figure 1-7

Figures 1-8 to 1-13 *These figures depict the spectrum of other causes of ophthalmia neonatorum.* ▶ *Figures 1-8 and 1-9 show primary herpes simplex virus (HSV) blepharoconjunctivokeratitis. Maculovesicular pustular lid and periorbital inflammatory reactions are evident. The cornea in Fig. 1-10 shows a hazy epithelium with peripheral corneal fluorescein staining, depicting associated corneal infection by HSV. Figure 1-11 shows diffuse conjunctival hyperemia without corneal involvement characteristic of "chemical conjunctivitis" associated with silver nitrate drops. Figure 1-12 shows conjunctival vesicles and peripheral corneal involvement from acute* Vaccinia *infection. Figure 1-13 shows diffuse corneal infiltration, edema, and scarring after a "ring" ulcer due to* Pseudomonas aeruginosa *bacterial infection.*

NEONATAL EYE DISEASE

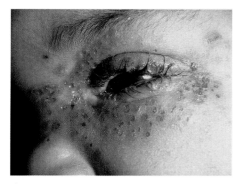

Figure 1-8

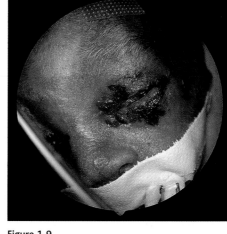

Figure 1-9

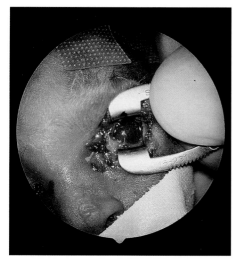

Figure 1-10

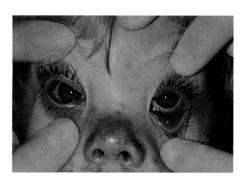

Figure 1-11

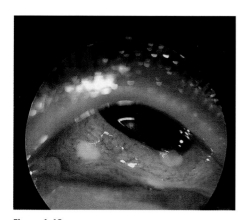

Figure 1-12

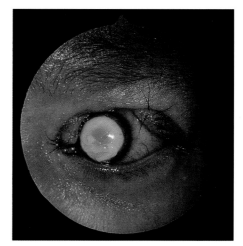

Figure 1-13

SELECTED REFERENCES

Barton LL: Povidone-iodine to prevent ophthalmia neonatorum [letter; comment]. N Engl J Med 333(2):127, 1995.

1989 Sexually transmitted diseases treatment guidelines: extracted from the Centers for Disease Control Guidelines [see comments]. *Pediatr Infect Dis J* 9(6):379–382; discussion 382–384, 1990.

1992 Update on the periodic medical examination. 4. Prophylaxis of gonococcal and Chlamydia ophthalmia in the newborn. Canadian study group on the periodic medical examination]. *Union Med Can* 122(6): 406–410, 1993.

Blanchard TJ, Mabey DC: Chlamydial infections. *Br J Clin Pract* 48(4):201–205, 1994.

Chandler JW, Rapoza PA: Ophthalmia neonatorum. *Int Ophthalmol Clin* 30(1):36–38, 1990.

Czajkowski J et al: Report of the commission for the prophylaxis of anterior segment eye infections newborns. *Ginekol Pol* 67(8): 421–422, 1996.

de Toledo AR, Chandler JW: Conjunctivitis of the newborn. *Infect Dis Clin North Am* 6(4):807–813, 1992.

De Schryver A, Meheus A: Epidemiology of sexually transmitted diseases: the global picture. *Bull World Health Org* 68(5):639–654, 1990.

Hammerschlag MR: Neonatal conjunctivitis. *Pediatr Ann* 22(6):346–351, 1993.

Hertle RW, Schaffer DB: Ophthalmia neonatorum: a clinical update. *Curr Concepts Ophthalmol* 3:39–47, 1995.

Isenberg SJ, Apt L, Wood M: A controlled trial of povidone-iodine as prophylaxis against ophthalmia neonatorum [see comments]. *N Engl J Med,* 332(9):562–566, 1995.

Mani VR, Vidya KC: A microbiological study of ophthalmia neonatorum in hospital-born babies. *J Indian Med Assoc* 95(7):416–417, 1997.

O'Hara MA: Ophthalmia neonatorum. *Pediatr Clin North Am* 40(4):715–725, 1993.

Oriel JD: Eminent venereologists 5: Carl Crede. *Genitourin Med* 67(1):67–69, 1991.

van Bogaert LJ: Ophthalmia neonatorum revisited. *Afr J Reprod Health* 2(1):81–86, 1998.

Whitcher JP: Neonatal ophthalmia: have we advanced in the last 20 years? *Int Ophthalmol Clin* 30(1):39–41, 1990.

CHAPTER 2

TORCH SYNDROMES

DAVID B. SCHAFFER

DEFINITION OF TERMS

Classically, the term *TORCH syndromes* referred to the congenital infections of toxoplasmosis, rubella, cytomegalic inclusion disease (CID), and herpes simplex virus. However, today it is a general term more widely used for any of the various known infectious agents that result in somewhat characteristic congenital diseases, which include syphilis, chickenpox, and acquired immunodeficiency syndrome (AIDS). Systemic and ocular findings may include both structural malformations and inflammatory processes, and although the ocular findings may be suggestive of a particular agent, the pathology seen can be so strikingly similar that the diagnosis cannot be made from the eye findings alone.

DIFFERENTIAL DIAGNOSIS

1. Congenital infection
2. Genetic ocular malformation
3. Intrauterine or birth canal trauma
4. Acquired neonatal infection

WORKUP

1. Family history for similar findings
2. Maternal history for symptoms during pregnancy
3. Careful systemic examination of newborn to delineate all abnormalities
4. Complete ophthalmologic examination
5. Viral cultures from urine, blood leukocytes, nasopharynx, skin lesions, maternal milk or cervical excretions, and any involved organ

6. Electron microscopic exam of urine or tissue for intranuclear and intracytoplasmic inclusions
7. Serologic tests from infant and mother (complement fixation; fluorescence assays; indirect or latex hemagglutination tests; enzyme-linked immunosorbent assay (ELISA) technique for cytomegalovirus (CMV)-specific IgM

TREATMENT (See Table 2-1 on page 10)

1. Systemic, agent-specific antibiotic, antifungal, or antiviral drug therapy
2. Local antiviral drug therapy (e.g., herpes simplex)
3. Occasionally, local cycloplegics and steroids (e.g., treatment of anterior uveitis)
4. Early surgical intervention (e.g., congenital cataracts, glaucoma)

CONCLUSIONS

Although some of the congenital infections are now rare (rubella, syphilis, chickenpox), some are still prevalent (CID, toxoplasmosis) and others are being discovered and are on the rise (AIDS). The ophthalmologist's role is to delineate and treat the eye findings, but the diagnosis depends on the isolation of the offending agent or its identification by serologic tests. This is critical because there are now some specific therapies available for the systemic findings. In the neonatal period, treatment for TORCH syndromes is systemic, often having toxic side effects that have to be monitored and administered by neonatology, pediatrics, or infectious disease specialists.

Table 2-1   TREATMENT TABLE

Disease	Treatment
Syphilitic interstitial keratitis (see Figs. 2-2)	Systemic penicillin, topical cycloplegics, and steroid solutions
Rubella (see Figs. 2-5–2-12)	Supportive, congenital glaucoma surgery, early surgery for congenital cataracts
Congenital toxoplasmosis (see Figs. 2-13–2-17)	Neonatal period: Systemic pyrimethamine (Daraprim), sulfadiazine, trisulfapyrimidine, folinic acid Recurrent retinochoroiditis: pyrimethamine (Daraprim), sulfadiazine, trisulfapyrimidine, supplemental folinic acid or clindamycin
Cytomegalic inclusion disease (CID) (see Figs. 2-18–2-23)	Ganciclovir and foscarnet: For AIDS-associated CMV retinitis Protection and prevention: CMV immune globulin Cytogram: For use in transplant patients
Herpes simplex virus (see Figs. 2-24–2-27)	Local: Idoxyuridine 1.0%, vidarabine 3.0%, trifluorothymidine 1.0% Systemic: Vidarabine, acyclovir Prevention: Identify women at high risk to transmit virus; starting at 34–36 weeks' gestation, perform weekly cultures and/or perform cesarean c-section when culture is positive and before membranes rupture
Varicella zoster virus (see Figs. 2-28–2-30)	Immune globulin [varicella zoster immune globulin (VZIG)] has not been found to be effective. Investigational: Vidarabine and acyclovir.
Neonatal candidiasis (see Figs. 2-31–2-33)	Parenteral amphotericin B and 5-fluorocytosine

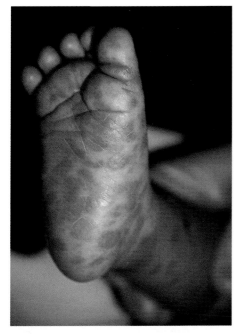

Figure 2-1

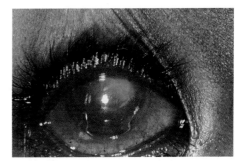

Figure 2-2

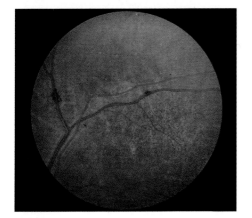

Figure 2-3

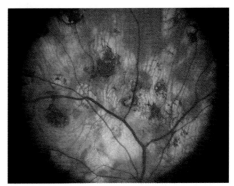

Figure 2-4

Figures 2-1 to 2-4 *These figures depict some of the systemic and ocular findings characteristic of congenital syphilis, which is caused by the bacterial spirochete* Treponema pallidum *and is now the least common of the classic TORCH syndromes. Figure 2-1 shows the typical maculopapular rash found on the soles of the feet, palms, trunk, and extremities. Acute interstitial keratitis (Fig. 2-2) is the most diagnostic eye finding, and occurs in 10% to 15% of infected infants. Figures 2-3 and 2-4 show a variety of chorioretinal lesions that are occasionally found at birth, but more often in later life.*

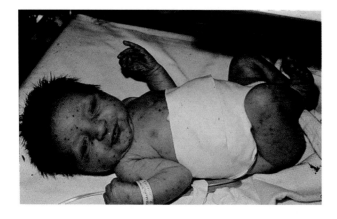

Figure 2-5

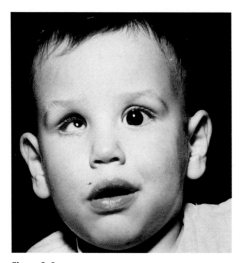

Figure 2-6

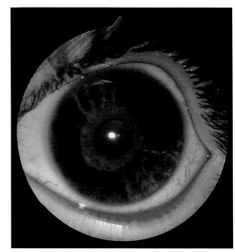

Figure 2-7

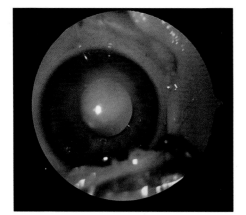

Figure 2-8

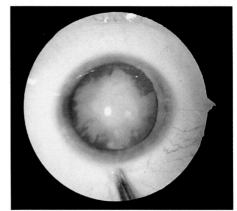

Figure 2-9

NEONATAL EYE DISEASE

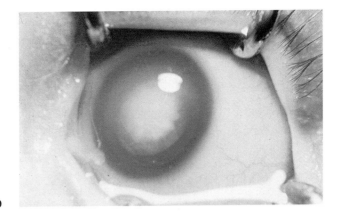

Figure 2-10

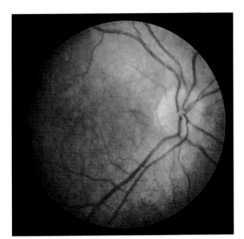

Figure 2-11

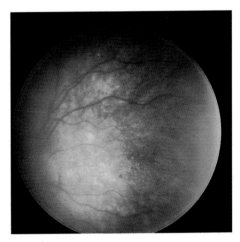

Figure 2-12

Figures 2-5 to 2-12 *These figures reveal some of the spectrum of the congenital rubella syndrome (CRS) caused by intracytoplasmic rubella virus, an RNA virus. The classic CRS triad includes heart, eye, and ear abnormalities and now occurs in only about 30 infants per year in the United States. Figure 2-5 reveals both the thrombocytopenic purpura and the classic morbilliform rash found at birth. Microphthalmia (Fig. 2-6) occurs in 20% of the involved infants who are infected early in the first trimester and can be unilateral or bilateral. Iris atrophy can involve the anterior stroma (Fig. 2-7) and the posterior pigment epithelium or the iris muscles and results in iris transillumination and poor dilatation. Cataracts, at least unilaterally, occur in about 50% of the infants, and with early first trimester involvement, bilateral cataracts have reportedly occurred in 75% of affected infants. The cataracts can be cortical and/or nuclear (Figs. 2-8 and 2-9), and often progress to morgagnian changes (Fig. 2-10). Figures 2-11 and 2-12 show variations of the "salt-and-pepper" pigmentary retinopathy that is the most common ocular finding in the CRS, occurring in up to 70% of involved neonates.*

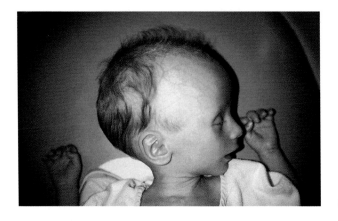

Figure 2-13

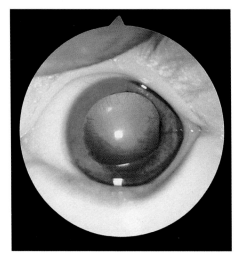

Figure 2-14

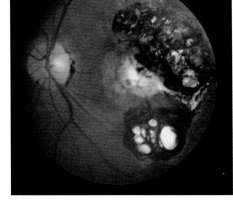

Figure 2-15

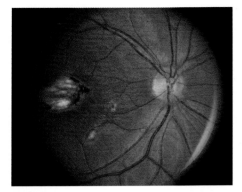

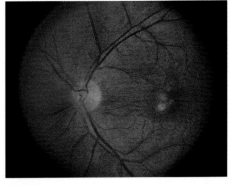

Figure 2-16   **Figure 2-17**

Figures 2-13 to 2-17   *These figures depict the spectrum of findings resulting from congenital toxoplasmosis, which results from the intrauterine infection by the protozoan* Toxoplasma gondii *and occurs in 1 to 2 per 1000 live births in the United States (about 3300 patients per year). The classic syndrome includes hydrocephaly (Fig. 2-13) with various degrees of mental retardation and/or seizures, retinochoroiditis, and randomly distributed intracranial calcifications. Acute (active) retinal lesions can present as leukokoria from massive exudative retinal and vitreous reactions (Fig. 2-14). The classic chorioretinal lesion (Fig. 2-15) is a large atrophic scar with varying degrees of atrophy, gliosis, and moderate to dense pigmentation. Recurrent or late attacks of retinochoroiditis (Figs. 2-16 and 2-17) are the most frequent sign of subclinical congenital toxoplasmosis, and may occur between 5 and 60 years of age, with a peak incidence in the teenage years.*

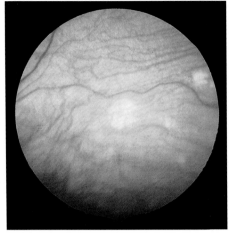

Figure 2-18

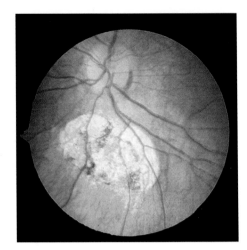

Figure 2-19

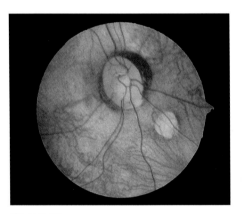

Figure 2-20

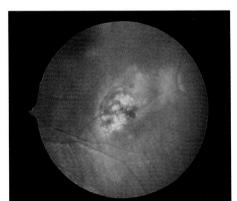

Figure 2-21

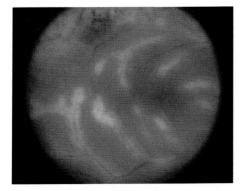

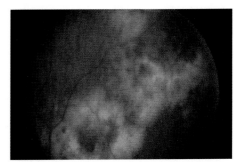

Figure 2-22   Figure 2-23

Figures 2-18 to 2-23   *These figures represent the reported and typical eye findings of congenital cytomegalic inclusion disease (CID), caused by the cytomegalovirus (CMV), a relatively large DNA virus in the herpesvirus family. It is now the leading cause of congenital infection in the United States, with an incidence of 0.5% to 2.4% of live births (average = 1/100; estimated to be about 33,000 instances per year). Most of the cases (90%) are subclinical, and 5% to 15% of patients with subclinical disease at birth will develop some sign of central nervous system (CNS) damage in childhood. Classic congenital CID consists of intrauterine growth retardation and prematurity, microcephaly, spastic diplegia, chorioretinal lesions, and periventricular intracranial calcifications. The most frequent ocular finding is chorioretinitis (Figs. 2-18 and 2-19), occurring in about 30% of overt congenital CID patients. The typical lesions are multiple, small, nonpigmented (Fig. 2-20), and often perivascular, and are associated with adjacent vessel sheathing. Full-thickness retinal necrosis results that is similar to and mimics toxoplasmosis or herpes simplex chorioretinitis (Fig. 2-21). Associated severe hemorrhaging and exudation may mimic a branched vein occlusion (Fig. 2-22), and when it is associated with acquired immunodeficiency syndrome (AIDS), a hemorrhagic vasculitis appearing like "pizza" (Fig. 2-23) may occur and results in retinal necrosis and scarring.*

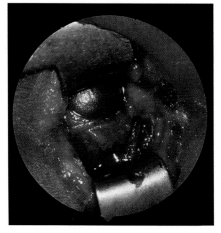

Figure 2-24

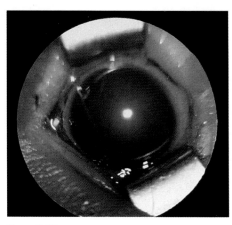

Figure 2-25

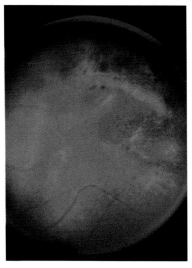

Figure 2-26

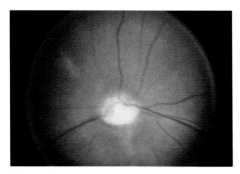

Figure 2-27

Figures 2-24 to 2-27 *These figures illustrate some of the ocular findings caused by herpes simplex virus (HSV). HSV is also a large DNA virus occurring in two types: HSV-1, which results in "cold sores" and involves the face and skin above the waist, and HSV-2, which has a genital distribution and causes 80% of the instances of congenital or neonatal disease. The disease is really neonatal, with only a few true congenital cases reported. It is estimated to occur in 1/2500 to 1/10,000 pregnancies per year in the United States, and the incidence is thought to be increasing. Of the cases, 33% to 90% are fatal and subclinical cases are rare. Ocular findings (neonatal and/or congenital) include conjunctivitis (herpetic ophthalmia neonatorum) that can be unilateral or bilateral and is characterized by lid edema, conjunctival chemosis and injection, and a serosanguineous discharge without follicular hypertrophy (Fig. 2-24). Without successful antiviral treatment, herpes keratitis may result, appearing as clouding of the cornea with diffuse superficial punctate keratitis (Fig. 2-25), dendritic and large geographic ulcers, stromal keratitis, or recurrent disciform keratitis. Chorioretinitis usually presents at 30 to 90 days, is usually an isolated finding, and only occasionally follows keratoconjunctivitis (Fig. 2-26). Optic nerve and retinal atrophy can be the end result of this infection (Fig. 2-27).*

NEONATAL EYE DISEASE

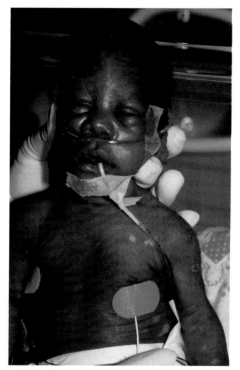

Figure 2-29

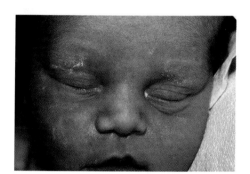

Figure 2-28

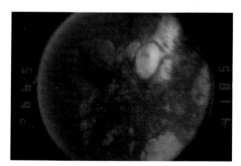

Figure 2-30

Figures 2-28 to 2-30 *These figures reveal some of the findings of congenital varicella (chicken-pox) infection caused by another member of the herpes simplex family, the varicella zoster virus (VZV). The congenital varicella embry-opathy or syndrome consists of scarring of the skin of the face (Fig. 2-28), body, and limbs (Fig. 2-29); microcephaly and cortical atro-phy; and lung, liver, and adrenal damage. The eye findings include microphthalmia, cataracts, anisocoria, Horner's syndrome, nonspecific chorioretinitis and optic atrophy, nystagmus, and strabismus (Fig. 2-30).*

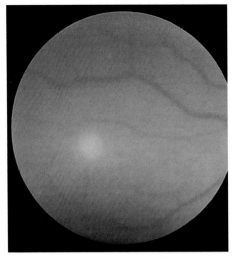

Figure 2-31

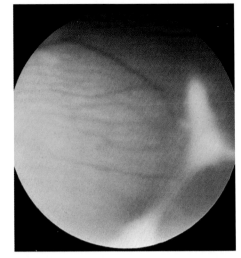

Figure 2-32

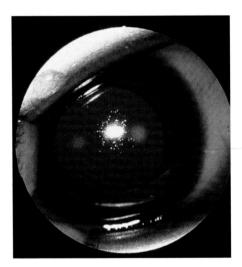

Figure 2-33

Figures 2-31 to 2-33 *These figures reveal the ocular findings of neonatal candidiasis, caused by the fungus* Candida albicans. *It is transmitted by an ascending vaginal disease penetrating intact membranes or chorioamnionitis with genital foreign bodies [cerclage or intrauterine device (IUD)]. The neonatal candidiasis syndrome includes the systemic findings of respiratory deterioration, erythematous burnlike dermatitis, temperature instability, generalized pustulosis, abdominal distention, guaiac-positive stools, carbohydrate intolerance, meningitis, and hypotension. The fungi are found in the blood, cerebrospinal fluid (CSF), and urine, and the infection is frequently fatal. The ocular findings are retinitis, vitriitis, and endophthalmitis, with the earliest lesions appearing as discrete, densely yellow-white opacities that mimic cotton-wool spots with overlying vitreous haze (Figs. 2-31 and 2-32). The lesions occur most often in the macular area, but they can be peripheral, and in later stages, white fungal "puffs" can be seen floating free in the vitreous (Fig. 2-33). (Figs. 2-31–2-33 courtesy of Earl A. Palmer, M.D.)*

NEONATAL EYE DISEASE

SELECTED REFERENCES

Edwards JE et al: Ocular manifestations of candida septicemia: review of seventy-six cases of hematogenous candida endophthalmitis. *Medicine (Balt)* 53:47–75, 1974.

Lambert SR, et al: Ocular manifestations of the congenital varicella syndrome. *Arch Ophthalmol* 107:52–56, 1989.

Palmer EA: Endogenous Candida endophthalmitis in infants. *Am J Ophthalmol* 89(3):388–395, 1980.

Plotkin SA et al: The congenital rubella syndrome in late infancy. *JAMA* 200:435–441, 1967.

Schaffer DB: Eye findings in intrauterine infections. *Clin Perinatol* 8:415–443, 1981.

Schaffer DB: Eye findings in neonates who have congenital infections: Part I. *J Calif Perinatal Assoc* 3:39–45, 1984.

Schaffer DB: Eye findings in neonates who have congenital infections: Part II. *J Calif Perinatal Assoc* 4:15–23, 1984.

Stagno S, et al: Herpesvirus infections of pregnancy. Part I: Cyto-megalovirus and Epstein-Barr virus infections. *N Engl J Med* 313:1270–1274, 1985.

CATARACTS AND DEVELOPMENTAL ANOMALIES OF THE LENS

WILLIAM MADIGAN III

DEFINITION OF TERMS

Light rays from objects in space are normally focused on the retina by both the cornea and the lens. A cataract is a lack of clarity in the crystalline lens. A cataract interferes with light passage from the environment to the retina, resulting in variable loss of some or all visual functions. Cataracts in the pediatric population can be present at birth or develop during childhood. Pediatric cataracts are most often of genetic origin and due to developmental anomalies of the lens fibers or metabolic disturbances. Adult cataracts are structurally different and usually the result of senescent changes occurring over many decades.

DIFFERENTIAL DIAGNOSIS

1. Sporadic or hereditary familial cataracts (Figs. 3-1–3-6)
2. Traumatic cataracts
3. Cataracts associated with a syndrome or a systemic disease (brief list) (Figs. 3-7–3-15)
   a. Craniofacial dysotoses: e.g., Crouzon's disease, Apert's syndrome
   b. Mandibulofacial syndromes: e.g., Hallermann-Streiff syndrome, Pierre Robin syndrome, Treacher Collins syndrome
   c. Skeletal syndromes: e.g., Conradi's syndrome, Marfan's syndrome, Albers-Schönberg disease, Weill-Marchesani syndrome, osteogenesis imperfecta
   d. Apical malformations: e.g., Laurence-Moon-Biedl syndrome, Meyer-Schwickerath syndrome, Rubinstein-Taybi syndrome
   e. CNS disease: e.g., Sjögren's syndrome, Marinesco-Sjögren syndrome
   f. Muscular disease: e.g., myotonic dystrophy
   g. Dermatologic disorders: e.g., congenital anhidrotic ectodermal dysplasia, Rothmund's syndrome, Schäfer's syndrome, congenital ichthyosis
   h. Chromosomal disorders: e.g., Down syndrome, Turner's syndrome, Patau's syndrome, Edward's syndrome
   i. Metabolic disturbances: e.g., galactosemia, galactose 1-phosphate uridyltransferase deficiency, galactokinase deficiency, abetalipoproteinemia, diabetes mellitus, Wilson's disease, Hurler's disease, Fabry's disease, cerebrotendinous xanthomatosis (cholestanolosis), Refsum's syndrome, mannosidosis, gyrate atrophy
4. Cataracts associated with other ocular diseases or anomalies: e.g., glaucoma, retinopathy of prematurity, uveitis (Figs. 3-16–3-20)
5. Cataracts associated with drugs or toxins: e.g., steroids, radiation
6. Cataracts associated with TORCH syndromes (see Chap. 2).

WORKUP

1. History
   a. Family and pregnancy: e.g., maternal infection, drug use, toxin exposure, or ionizing radiation; complications of pregnancy; birth weight; gestational age; Apgar scores
   b. Neonatal and infantile history; e.g., medication, illness, developmental milestones, pediatrician's report of development and growth
2. Patient examination, e.g., central, steady, and maintained (CSM) method for infants or preverbal children; subjective acuity measurement using illiterate E, HOTV, or other method; visual evoked potential, preferential looking techniques, pupils, external examination, motility examination, retinoscopy before and after dilation with a cycloplegic agent; slit lamp examination before and after dilation; fundus examination; ultrasonography; consultation with genetics service
3. Ophthalmic examination of siblings, parents, and parent's siblings as dictated by family history
4. Laboratory evaluation: The laboratory evaluation is dependent upon the type of cataract plus physical and development findings. General laboratory evaluation might include complete blood count (CBC), urine test for reducing substances and amino acid analysis; serum glucose, calcium, and phosphorus measurements; immunologic tests for TORCH; and enzyme essay for galactokinase and galactotransferase deficiency.

TREATMENT

Children are developing key neuronal connections (synaptogenesis) serving vision until at least the end of the first decade of life. Anything causing unequal or abnormal visual input during this time period (such as a cataract) will interfere with the neurodevelopment of vision (amblyopia). This amblyopia will result in irreversible loss of vision if not treated during infancy and childhood. Because of the unique sensitivity of the developing visual system, cataracts in children require urgent diagnosis and treatment, beginning with rapid referral to an eye-care specialist. Neonates born with visually significant cataracts typically have surgical removal of the lens during the first days or weeks of life to optimize visual outcomes. Surgical removal of the lens clears the visual axis, but equally important in the visual rehabilitation of the child is the replacement of the natural lens's focusing power. This is typically accomplished with glasses and/or extended-wear contact lenses for children under 2 years of age. Older children may be candidates for intraocular lens implants similar to those used in adults.

CONCLUSIONS

Visually significant cataracts in children are diagnosed and treated on an urgent basis. Rapid restoration of a clear visual axis with a focused retinal image is the goal. Early detection and referral together with modern techniques in surgery and optical rehabilitation have resulted in improved visual outcomes in the great majority of children.

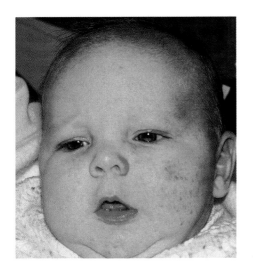

Figure 3-1 *This figure shows an asymmetric red reflex. The normal red reflex present in the left eye is absent in the right eye. Such a finding could be the sign of opacity somewhere in the visual axis and requires urgent eye-care evaluation.*

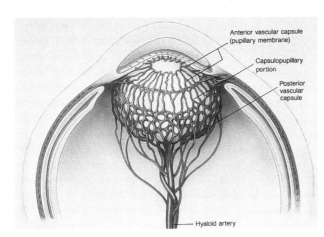

Anterior vascular capsule
(pupillary membrane)

Capsulopupillary
portion

Posterior
vascular
capsule

Hyaloid artery

Figure 3-2 *This embryologic illustration shows the lens, which is formed by surface ectoderm in the first trimester of life. It is surrounded by a basement membrane, the lens capsule, and is sequestered for the rest of the individual's life. Cortical fibers build around the central nucleus throughout early life, with sequential layers similar to those found in an onion. The location of the opacified lens fibers can give an indication as to when lens development was affected.*

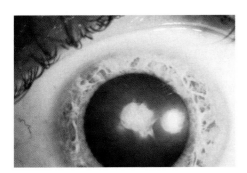

Figure 3-3 *This figure shows a* nuclear *cataract, implying disruption early in the lens development. Usually dense and affecting the central visual axis, these cataracts have an early and profound effect on visual development.*

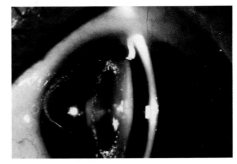

Figure 3-4 *This figure shows a* lamellar *cataract. Note that the central nucleus is clear and opacification is in the* outer *cortical fibers. This opacity occurred later in development.*

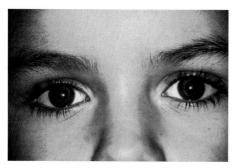

Figure 3-5 *This figure illustrates bilateral cataracts. These cataracts are more often associated with a smaller globe and are often heritable (54%), whereas unilateral cataracts are typically sporadic and nonheritable (94%).*

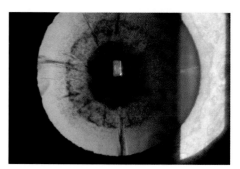

Figure 3-6 *This figure shows a complex cataract affecting both the nucleus and the peripheral lamellar layer.*

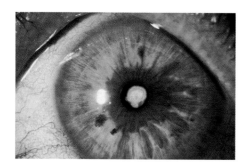

Figure 3-7 *This figure shows a typical* anterior polar *cataract. This type of cataract does not affect vision because it is distant from the nodal point of the eye where focused light converges en route to the retina. It is now recognized that these cataracts may enlarge over time and are associated with astigmatism in the eye, becoming visually significant.*

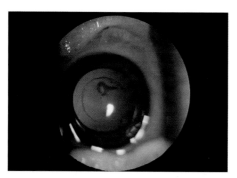

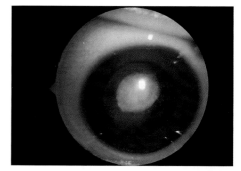

Figures 3-8 and 3-9 *These figures show a type of lens anomaly called* posterior lenticonus. *There is an area of missing lens capsule posteriorly that, over time, results in cortical fibers bowing out posteriorly into the vitreous. These fibers progressively opacify, requiring lens removal. This largely monocular condition has an excellent prognosis because the critical early stages of visual development occur normally, unlike with nuclear cataracts.*

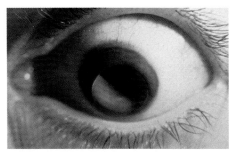
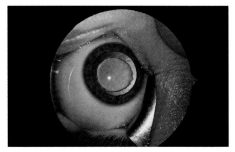

Figures 3-10 and 3-11 *These figures show the condition of* microspherophakia. *This small, round lens may dislocate into the anterior chamber of the eye in front of the iris, causing glaucoma. The lens can sometimes be stabilized in the proper location (behind the iris) by use of the miotic drop pilocarpine until an urgent ophthalmic exam is obtained.*

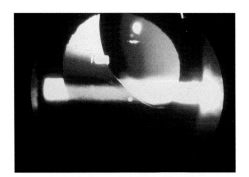
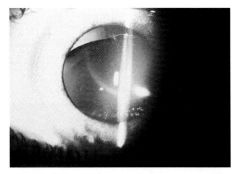

Figures 3-12 and 3-13 *These figures illustrate lens dislocations. Any disease causing loss of zonular support of the lens can cause its dislocation. As the lens shifts, increasing myopia and astigmatism are induced, eventually requiring lens removal. Figure 3-12 shows the typical superior temporal dislocation in a patient with Marfan's syndrome. Figure 3-13 shows the inferonasal displacement typical in patients with homocystinuria.*

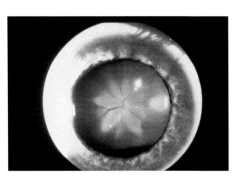
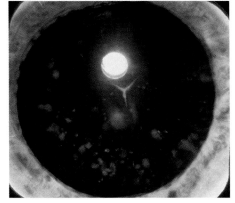

Figures 3-14 and 3-15 *These figures show a* sunflower *cataract (Fig. 3-14) and a punctate coronary cataract (Fig. 3-15), which are often a result of metabolic disturbances such as Wilson's disease and hypocalcemia.*

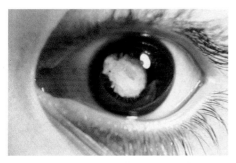

Figure 3-16 *This figure shows a complicated calcific cataract associated with persistent hyperplastic primary vitreous.*

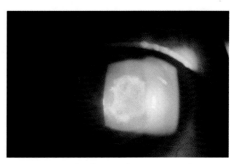

Figure 3-17 *This figure shows a* posterior subcapsular *cataract. This cataract is typically associated with intraocular inflammation and chronic use of steroids.*

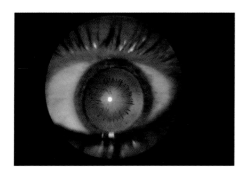

Figure 3-18

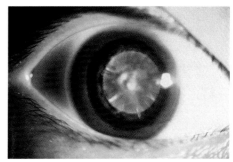

Figure 3-19

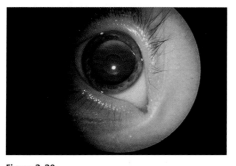

Figure 3-20

Figures 3-18 to 3-20 *These figures show the* lamellar *(oil-droplet) cataracts associated with galactosemia (Figs. 3-18, 3-19) and Zellweger (cerebrohepatorenal) syndrome (Fig. 3-20).*

SELECTED REFERENCES

Bateman JR: Genetics in pediatric ophthalmology. *Pediatr Clin North Am* 30:1015, 1983.

Cavallaro BE et al: Posterior chamber intraocular use in children. *J Pediatr Ophthalmol Strabismus* 35:254–263, 1998.

Dutton J, Slamovitis T (eds): Viewpoints: Visual rehabilitation in aphakic children. *Surv Ophthalmol* 34:365–384, 1990.

Gordon T, Donzis P: Refractive development of the human eye. *Arch Ophthalmol* 104:651–652, 1985.

Rahi JS, Dezateux C: Congenital and infantile cataract in the United Kingdom: underlying or associated factors. *Invest Ophthalmol Vis Sci* 41(8):2108–2114, 2000.

Spierer A, Desatnik H, Blumenthal M: Secondary cataract in infants after extracapsular cataract extraction and anterior vitrectomy. *Ophthalmic Surg* 23:625–627, 1992.

Taylor D (ed.): *Paediatric Ophthalmology*, 2nd ed. Blackwell Scientific, Malden, MA, pp 445–476, 1998.

Vaegan TD: Critical period for deprivation amblyopia in children. *Trans Ophthalmol Soc UK* 99:432, 1979.

CHAPTER 4

GLAUCOMA AND DEVELOPMENTAL ABNORMALITIES OF THE ANTERIOR SEGMENT

RICHARD W. HERTLE

DEFINITION OF TERMS

Developmental diseases of the cornea and anterior segment of the eye usually result in clinically significant structural changes and almost
always affect vision. Loss of vision is often due
to a combination of amblyopia and obstruction
of the visual axis. These diseases are usually
differentiated based on those that remain stable
(dysgenesis) and those that progress (dystrophies). They are usually diagnosed shortly after
birth or within the first year of life. They can be
inherited due to sporadic gene and chromosome
abnormalities or be the result of metabolic diseases. Bilateral developmental diseases of the
anterior segment are often associated with systemic syndromes. The structures of the anterior
segment (cornea, trabeculum, iris, and lens) can
be involved in isolation or in various combinations.

DIFFERENTIAL DIAGNOSIS

1. Glaucoma—Congenital and juvenile glaucoma are infrequent but caused by over 50
   primary and secondary mechanisms.
   Infants will present with tearing, blepharospasm, photophobia, and large, cloudy
   corneas. These children need prompt ophthalmic evaluation because surgical treatment is almost always necessary (Figs.
   4-1–4.5).
2. Corneal dermoid—A dermoid is a benign
   choristoma composed of both skinlike neu-

roectodermal tissue and mesodermal elements. Typical components of dermoids
include hair follicles and adipose tissue.
Most dermoids are solid, but some lesions
of this type are cystic. The most common
ocular site for dermoid lesions is the limbus
inferotemporally (Figs. 4-6–4-8).
3. Sclerocornea and cornea plana—This form
   of anterior segment dysgenesis is due to
   poor differentiation of the cornea from the
   sclera. The cornea is opaque, flat, and
   small. An opaque cornea and associated
   retinal and optic nerve anomalies often
   limit vision (Figs. 4-9–4-11).
4. Congenital corneal anomalies—The normal newborn cornea is about 9.5 to 10 mm
   in horizontal length, reaching an adult size
   of about 12.0 mm by 2 years of age. Abnormalities of corneal size and shape in childhood include megalocornea, keratoglobus,
   keratoconus, and microcornea (Figs. 4-14
   and 4-15).
5. Anterior segment dysgenesis—These are a
   spectrum of developmental disturbances of
   the cornea, trabeculum, iris, and lens, all of
   which have in common the possible clinical
   consequence of glaucoma and opacity of the
   visual axis. These disturbances include posterior embryotoxon, Axenfeld-Reiger syndrome, posterior keratoconus, and Peter's
   anomaly (Figs. 4-12, 4-13, 4-16–4-20).
6. Metabolic disease—There are numerous
   corneal manifestations of metabolic disease. They can result in various combinations of corneal opacification, abnormal

material deposition, erosion, edema, thinning, and neovascularization. More common systemic diseases include tyrosinemia, cystinosis, dyslipoproteinemias, lysosomal storage disease, gout, Wilson's disease, hemochromatosis, and amlyoidosis.

7. Aniridia and iris coloboma—This is a panocular, bilateral, developmental disorder where there is little to no iris tissue. A defect in the PAX6 gene on chromosome 11 is responsible for this condition. The familial form is autosomal dominant, but a third of cases are sporadic. The sporadic form is more commonly associated with Wilm's tumor and mental retardation (ARG) [Miller's Syndrome: aniridia–Wilm's tumor, retardation, genitourinary abnormalities (triad)]. Other eye findings include decreased vision, nystagmus, foveal hypoplasia, cataract, glaucoma, corneal pannus, and high refractive errors. Iris colobomas are "typical" if they occur in the inferonasal quadrant. They are explained by failure of fusion of the embryonic fissure in the fifth week of gestation. They are often associated with other ocular and systemic diseases, e.g., trisomy 13, triploidy, 4p–, 11q–, 18r, trisomy 18, and Coloboma, Heart defects, Atresia of chonae, Retarded growth & devel., Genital hypoplasia, Ear anomolies and/or hearing loss (CHARGE) syndrome (Figs. 4-21–4-23).

8. Corneal dystrophies—These are bilateral, symmetric, inherited conditions that begin early in life. Most are slowly progressive, and many can lead to vision loss and painful corneal edema or recurrent erosions. They are classified largely on the basis of a predominant layer of corneal involvement and appearance, although new classification schemes also incorporate heredity, genetics, and histopathology. Corneal dystrophies include the anterior dystrophies such as anterior basement membrane dystrophy, juvenile epithelial dystrophy, and Reis-Bucklers dystrophy.

The stromal dystrophies include granular, macular, lattice, gelatinous droplike, Schnyder's central crystalline, fleck, and central cloudy. The endothelial dystrophies include Fuchs, posterior polymorphous, and congenital hereditary endothelial. The ectactic dystrophies include keratoconus, keratoglobus, and pellucid marginal degeneration (Figs. 4-24–4-28).

WORKUP

1. Complete history (pregnancy, labor, delivery, growth and development)
2. Associated systemic conditions
3. Family history
4. Ophthalmic evaluation (under anesthesia if necessary)
5. Genetic consultation (as necessary)
6. Specific laboratory testing (e.g., metabolic diseases)

TREATMENT

1. Treat underlying condition (e.g., reduce pressure in glaucoma)
2. Clear visual axis (medically or surgically)
3. Treat associated amblyopia
4. Treat associated refractive errors and strabismus

CONCLUSIONS

The child presenting with an obviously malformed anterior segment (cornea, iris, lens) presents diagnostic and clinical treatment challenges. These diseases require the full knowledge, investigative capabilities, and modern technologic advances of the eye-care profession. It is only through prompt diagnosis and treatment that children with these disorders may regain or retain useful vision.

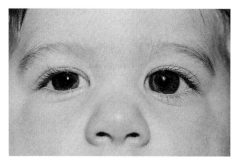

Figure 4-1

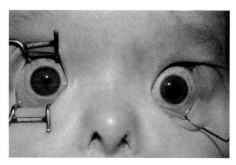

Figure 4-2

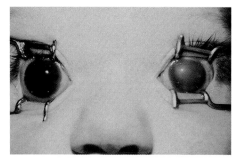

Figure 4-3

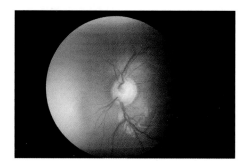

Figure 4-4

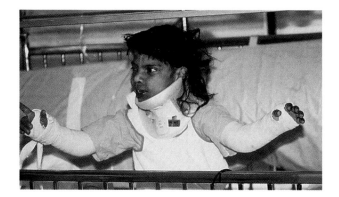

Figure 4-5

Figures 4-1 to 4-5 *These figures show the clinical appearance of children with congenital glaucoma or* buphthalmos. *These children usually present between 2 and 12 months of age with tearing, photophobia, blepharospasm, and corneal enlargement and clouding. Figure 4-1 illustrates an infant with unilateral corneal enlargement and no significant difference in the clarity of the involved left cornea. Figure 4-2 shows a child with oculo-facial-digital syndrome, bilateral microphthalmia, and cloudy corneas due to associated glaucoma. Figure 4-3 shows the typical appearance of bilateral bupthalmos and cloudy corneas associated with congenital glaucoma. Figure 4-4 shows the atrophic, cupped optic nerve of a child with congenital glaucoma. Figure 4-5 shows a child needing temporary restraints to protect her eye after glaucoma surgery. She has developmental delay and congenital glaucoma associated with congenital maramata marginata telan-giectasia and is self-abusive.*

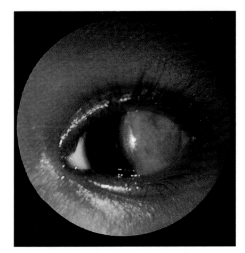

Figure 4-6

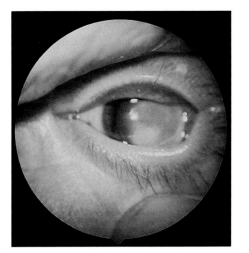

Figure 4-7

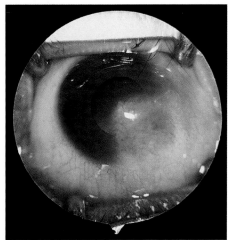

Figure 4-8

Figures 4-6 to 4-8 *These are photographs of typical dermoid tumors of the cornea. These choristomas can appear fleshy, white, elevated, or flat and can often have visible hairs or cilia protruding from them. They can affect vision by causing severe refractive errors and by direct obstruction of the visual axis.*

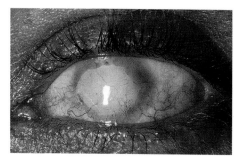

Figure 4-9

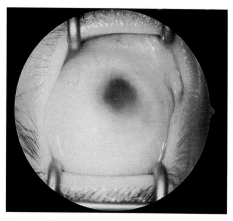

Figure 4-10

Figures 4-9 to 4-11 *These figures illustrate the varied appearance of sclerocornea. Figure 4-9 shows scleralization of a large portion of the central cornea with abundant corneal vascularization. Sclerocornea is often associated with microphthalmos and cornea plana ("flat") (Fig. 4-10). Figure 4-11 shows peripheral sclerocornea with vascularization and associated central haze due to less severe central corneal involvement.*

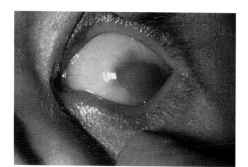

Figure 4-11

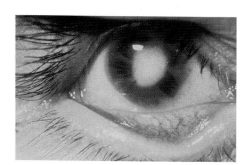

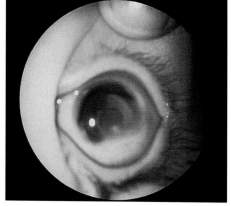

Figures 4-12 and 4-13 *These figures show a severe form of anterior segment dysgenesis called* Peter's anomaly. *Figure 4-12 shows a central corneal leukoma, iris strands attached to a posterior corneal defect, iris atrophy and/or dysplasia, and glaucoma. Figure 4-13 shows Peter's anomaly associated with iris aplasia, sclerocornea, microphthalmos, and cataract.*

GLAUCOMA AND DEVELOPMENTAL ABNORMALITIES OF THE ANTERIOR SEGMENT

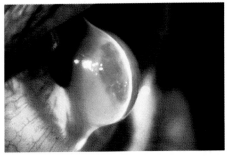 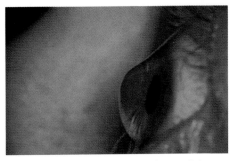

Figures 4-14 and 4-15 *The cornea can be involved in a congenital dystrophy called keratoglobus where the tissue is thinned and protruding, often with vascularization and corneal clouding (Fig. 4-14). A dystrophic process such as osteogenesis imperfecta can also cause keratoglobus (Fig. 4-15).*

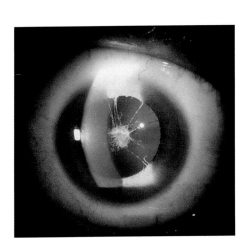 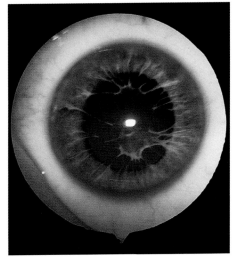

Figures 4-16 and 4-17 *The iris can be the predominant structure involved in anterior segment dysgenesis. Figures 4-16 and 4-17 show persistent fetal vasculature as "iris strands," which are often attached to the anterior lens capsule. These are most commonly not visually disabling but can be associated with cataract or other angle anomalies leading to glaucoma.*

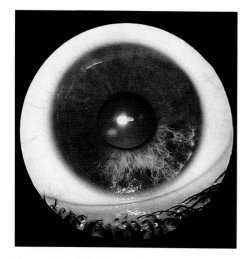

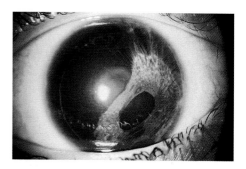

Figure 4-18 *This figure shows congenital, segmental iris hypoplasia without other ocular disease. This iris condition can also be seen after trauma and ocular herpes zoster infection.*

Figure 4-19 *This eye has severe iris hypoplasia and correctopia associated with the irido-corneo-endothelial (ICE) syndrome. This is highly associated with the development of glaucoma.*

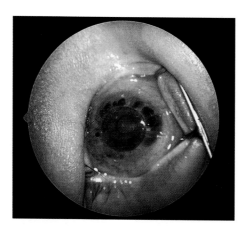

Figure 4-20 *This eye has severe anterior segment dysgenesis and has had a successful corneal transplant.*

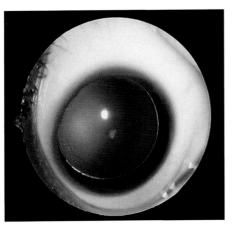

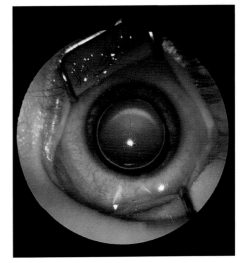

Figures 4-21 and 4-22 *These eyes show the varied appearance of the iris associated with aniridia. There is almost complete absence of the iris in Fig. 4-21, but aniridia eyes often have some iris present (Fig. 4-22). Other eye findings with aniridia include glaucoma, corneal pannus, cataract, foveal hypoplasia, and nystagmus. The sporadic form can be associated with a Wilm's tumor, although this finding is not seen in the familial form of aniridia.*

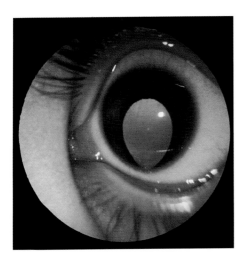

Figure 4-23 *The iris of this eye has a typical inferior nasal defect associated with an iris coloboma. This can be associated with colobomatous malformations of the ciliary body, choroid, retina, and optic nerve.*

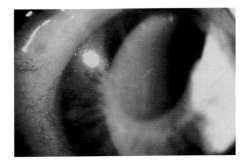

Figure 4-24 *This cornea shows linear, maplike fluorescein staining of the epithelium typical of anterior basement membrane dystrophy. Patients with this dystrophy suffer from repeated painful corneal erosions.*

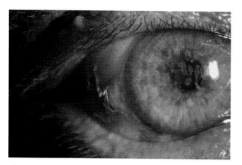 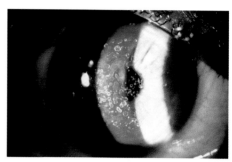

Figures 4-25 and 4-26 *Granular degeneration. These corneas have* granular *deposits of hyaline degeneration with distinct borders within the corneal stroma. This bilateral, autosomal dominant degeneration can occasionally cause visual symptoms and lead to recurrent corneal erosions.*

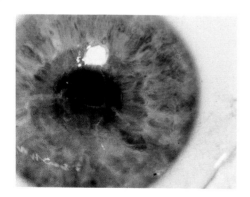 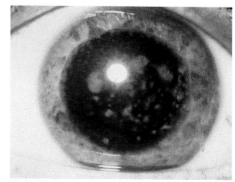

Figure 4-27 *Lattice degeneration. This cornea has* lattice *deposits of amyloidlike material within the entire corneal stroma. This bilateral, autosomal dominant degeneration leads to severe vision loss and painful recurrent corneal erosions.*

Figure 4-28 *Macular degeneration. This cornea has grayish, opaque spots with indistinct borders due to a local keratocyte mucopolysaccharidosis. This bilateral, autosomal recessive degeneration leads to vision loss and mild recurrent erosive symptoms.*

SELECTED REFERENCES

Beauchamp GR: Anterior segment dysgenesis keratolenticular adhesion and aniridia. *J Pediatr Ophthalmol Strabismus* 17(1):55–58, 1980.

Churchill A, Booth A. Genetics of aniridia and anterior segment dysgenesis. *Br J Ophthalmol* 80(7):669–673, 1996.

Craig JE, Mackey DA: Glaucoma genetics: Where are we? Where will we go? *Curr Opin Ophthalmol* 10(2):126–134, 1999.

deLuise VP, Anderson DR: Primary infantile glaucoma (congenital glaucoma). *Survey Ophthalmology* 28(1):1–19, 1983.

Hittner HM et al: Variable expressivity of autosomal dominant anterior segment mesenchymal dysgenesis in six generations. *Am J Ophthalmol* 93(1):57–70, 1982.

Mandal AK, Naduvilath TJ, Jayagandan A: Surgical results of combined trabeculotomy-trabeculectomy for developmental glaucoma. *Ophthalmology* 105(6):974–982, 1998.

Pernoud FG 3d: Inherited and developmental corneal disorders. *Pediatr Ann* 19(5): 326–333, 1990.

Sarfarazi M: Recent advances in molecular genetics of glaucomas. *Hum Mol Genet* 6(10):1667–1677, 1997.

Traboulsi EI: Ocular malformations and developmental genes. *J Pediatr Ophthalmol Strabismus* 2(6):317–323, 1998.

Williams DL: A comparative approach to anterior segment dysgenesis. *Eye* 7(Pt 5):607–616, 1993.

CONGENITAL ANOMALIES OF THE LIDS AND ORBIT

JOHN T. TONG and JILL A. FOSTER

DEFINITION OF TERMS

PUNCTAL ANOMALIES AND FISTULAS

Congenital anomalies of the puncta of the naso-lacrimal drainage system include absence, imperforation (Figs. 5-1 and 5-2) and duplication (Figs. 5-3 and 5-4). These may involve either the upper or lower puncta, or both. An absent punctum may be associated with an absent canaliculus. A thin membrane is seen with an imperforate punctum. Punctal agenesis or dysgenesis may be suspected if epiphora is present without significant mucopurulent discharge. Inspection of the lid will reveal this abnormality.

LID COLOBOMAS

An eyelid coloboma is a clefting defect that forms a notch involving the eyelid margin. If it occurs in the upper eyelid, it tends to affect the medial half (Fig. 5-5) and is usually an isolated event, although it may sometimes be seen with other conditions (Fig. 5-6), such as Goldenhar's syndrome.

EPICANTHAL FOLDS

Epicanthal fold, or canthal webbing, describes the fold of skin that extends from the eyelid to the medial canthus. Different names are given to the different types of folds seen, depending upon where the fold originates (Figs. 5-7 and 5-8). Epicanthus palpebralis appears to originate equally from both the upper and lower eyelids and is the most common type. Epicanthus tarsalis appears to originate from the upper eyelid and is commonly seen in Asians. Epicanthal folds may sometimes give the appearance that the child's eyes are esotropic even though they are not (pseudostrabismus). Epicanthus inversus appears to originate from the lower eyelid and may be seen with the blepharophimosis syndrome.

LID MALPOSITIONS

Eyelid retraction occurs when the resting position of the eyelid is either higher (upper eyelid) or lower (lower eyelid) than its normal position. Although the etiology is unknown, upper eyelid retraction is a common finding in neonates. Eyelid retraction may occur without any cause or may be associated with other conditions such as neonatal Graves' disease, hydrocephalus, dorsal midbrain disease, and levator fibrosis.

Congenital entropion occurs when the eyelid margin turns inward. It typically involves the lower eyelid, less commonly the upper eyelid. When the eyelid margin and eyelashes rub against the eye, disruption of the corneal epithelium with subsequent infection and scarring may result. Epiblepharon occurs when a horizontal fold of skin and orbicularis muscle extends over the eyelid crease. This may cause a mechanical entropion of the eyelid margin.

Congenital ectropion (Fig. 5-9) occurs when the eyelid margin turns outward. It may be seen with either the upper or lower eyelids. This may be accompanied by eyelid retraction or vertical shortening of the eyelid. Congenital ectropion may be associated with other conditions, such as blepharophimosis and Down's syndrome.

Blepharophimosis syndrome is characterized by a shortened horizontal width of the palpebral fissure, ptosis, telecanthus, and epicanthus inversus. It is inherited in an autosomal dominant manner, although many cases are also sporadic.

ANOPHTHALMIA

True anophthalmia is very rare. Typically, tiny remnants of the eye are noted on pathologic evaluation even when there is no grossly visible globe (Fig. 5-10). *Clinical anophthalmia* is the term used to describe this condition. Unilateral anophthalmia or microphthalmia may be associated with structural abnormalities of the contralateral eye. Without the stimulus of a normally growing globe, the growth of the bony orbit and soft tissue adnexa is stunted. This also results in ipsilateral midface hypoplasia.

MICROPHTHALMIA

Microphthalmia describes a congenitally small eye and occurs on a continuum with anophthalmia. The structures of the eye may be normal or severely affected. It is usually unilateral (Figs. 5-11 to 5-13), although rarely it can affect both eyes. Although the microphthalmic eye often has a small cornea, microcornea can occur without microphthalmia and microphthalmia may rarely occur without microcornea. It may also be associated with glaucoma, Peter's anomaly, cataracts, persistent hyperplastic vitreous, colobomas, and retinal problems. One form of microphthalmia is microphthalmia with orbital cyst. This presents with a progressively enlarging mass. The microphthalmic eye itself may be hidden from view.

ANKYLOBLEPHARON

Ankyloblepharon is the partial or complete fusion of the epithelial edge of the eyelid margins (Fig. 5-14). During fetal development, the eyelids are naturally fused until the seventh month of gestation. A maturational failure may leave the eyelids partially or completely fused at the time of birth.

CRYPTOPHTHALMIA

In Cryptophthalmos the eyelid structures never form, so there is a continuum between the epithelium of the face and the surface of the cornea. This condition occurs when there is anomalous or inadequate migration of the epithelial eyelid folds. The mesenchyme does not completely invaginate the lid fold, and the eye epithelializes without an eyelid covering. Part or all of the eyebrow, eyelashes, eyelid, palpebral fissure, and conjunctiva may be missing. The eye itself may be microphthalmic, and severe defects in the eye are usually found (Figs. 5-15 and 5-16).

CYCLOPIA AND SYNOPHTHALMIA

Cyclopia is a complete fusion of the two globes into one, whereas synophthalmia is a partial fusion. Synophthalmia occurs more frequently (Fig. 5-17). In both cases, the eye is situated in a midline orbit. With cyclopia (Fig. 5-18), there is often an absence of the retinal ganglion cells and optic nerve. The optic chiasm is missing, and there is severe failure of midline differentiation of the brain that is incompatible with life. A proboscis is found superior to the eye. Some cases are associated with chromosomal abnormalities, such as trisomy 13.

WORKUP

1. Full family, maternal, and child history
2. Full ophthalmic evaluation
3. Possible genetics evaluation
4. Possible craniofacial team evaluation
5. Orbital imaging (CAT scan, MRI)

TREATMENT

1. Epiphora—Topical antibiotics, massage, probing, and surgical reconstruction of the nasolacrimal system
2. Eyelid coloboma—Lubrication, surgical repair
3. Epicanthal folds—Surgical modification
4. Congenital entropion or ectropion—Observation and lubrication, surgical repair
5. Epiblepharon—Surgical reconstruction
6. Blepharophimosis—Surgical reconstruction
7. Ankyloblepharon—Surgical reconstruction
8. Anophthalmia or microphthalmia—Stimulating bony orbital growth with the placement of static orbital implants or hydrophilic or injectable orbital expanders.

In addition, soft tissue growth is important to allow the retention of a prosthesis. Management of the microphthalmia depends upon the visual potential of the eye. If there is potential, then glasses and/or amblyopia treatment may be needed. In an eye with no visual potential, a cosmetic shell or contact lens may be fitted over the eye.

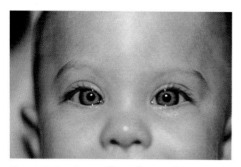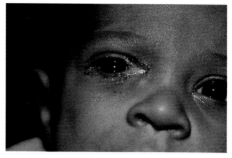

Figures 5-1 and 5-2 *These figures show two infants with epiphora (Fig. 5-1) and mucoid discharge (Fig. 5-2) due to nasolacrimal duct obstruction. This is usually due to an imperforate end of the nasolacrimal system in the nose.*

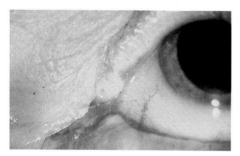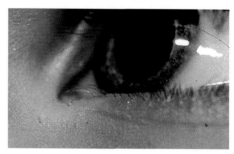

Figures 5-3 and 5-4 *These figures show duplication of the upper puncta (Fig. 5-3) and a fistula to the medial canthal skin (Fig. 5-4), both of which are congenital developmental abnormalities of the upper nasolacrimal system.*

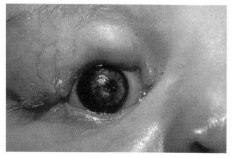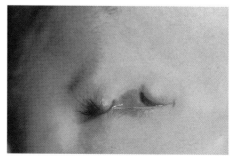

Figures 5-5 and 5-6 *Fig. 5-5 and Fig. 5-6 show a congenital absence of the middle portion of the upper lid called an eyelid coloboma. The lid skin can be fused with the eye (Fig. 5-6) and be associated with other eye abnormalities. Severe exposure keratitis can result if the lid does not protect the surface of the eye.*

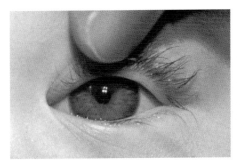

Figure 5-7

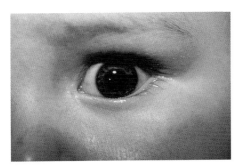

Figure 5-8

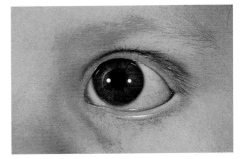

Figure 5-9

Figures 5-7 to 5-9 *These figures show congenital lid malpositions. Increased epicanthal folds are seen inferiorly in Fig. 5-7 and superiorly in Fig. 5-8. Figure 5-9 shows congenital ectropion of the lower lid.*

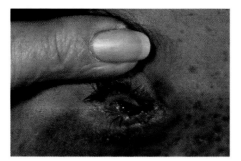

Figure 5-10

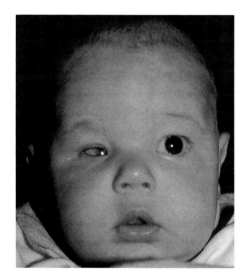

Figure 5-11

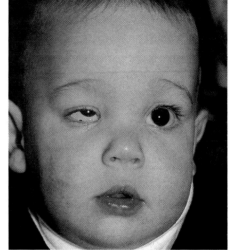

Figure 5-12

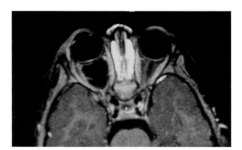

Figure 5-13

Figures 5-10 to 5-13 *These figures show the clinical spectrum of anophthalmia and microphthalmia. Figure 5-10 shows an anophthalmic orbit, whereas Figs. 5-11 and 5-12 show an example of unilateral microphthalmia. Figure 5-13 shows a CAT scan of the orbit of a patient with unilateral microphthalmia with a congenital cyst of the globe (seen in the posterior orbit).*

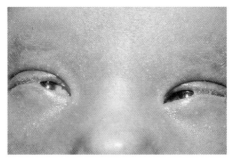

Figure 5-14 *This figure shows a child with bilateral ankyloblepharon (fusion) of the eyelids.*

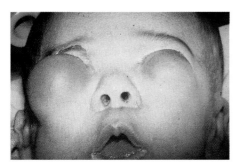 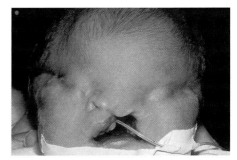

Figures 5-15 and 5-16 *These figures show the spectrum of congenital cryptophthalmos. Figure 5-15 shows an infant with bilateral cystic microphthalmos and cryptophthalmos, and Fig. 5-16 shows an infant with Fraser's syndrome with severe midfacial clefting, hypertelorism, cystic microphthalmos, and cryptophthalmos.*

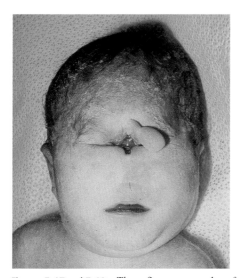 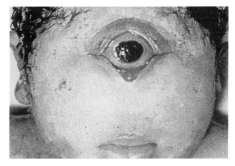

Figures 5-17 and 5-18 *These figures examples of cyclopia and synophthalmia with the fused proboscis to the maldeveloped, synophthalmic orbits in Fig. 5-17, and no proboscis in the infant with a more typical "cyclopia" pictured in Fig. 5-18.*

Agashe AP et al: Fraser's syndrome. *J Postgrad Med* 38(4):208–210, 1992.

Bacal DA et al: Ankyloblepharon filiforme adnatum in trisomy 18. *J Pediatr Ophthalmol Strabismus* 30(5):337–339, 1993.

Crawford JS: Congenital eyelid anomalies in children. *J Pediatr Ophthalmol Strabismus* 21(4):140–149, 1984.

Hornby SJ et al: Regional variation in blindness in children due to microphthalmos, anophthalmos and coloboma. *Ophthalmic Epidemiol* 7(2):127–138, 2000.

Jacquemin C, Mullaney PB, Bosley TM: Ophthalmological and intracranial anomalies in patients with clinical anophthalmos. *Eye* 14(Pt 1):82–87, 2000.

Shields SR: Managing eye disease in primary care. Part 2. How to recognize and treat common eye problems. *Postgrad Med* 108(5):83–86, 91–96, 2000.

Walton WT, Enzenauer RW, Cornell FM: Abortive cryptophthalmos: a case report and a review of cryptophthalmos. *J Pediatr Ophthalmol Strabismus* 27(3):129–132, 1990.

Yeo LM, Willshaw HE: Large congenital upper lid coloboma—successful delayed conservative management. *J Pediatr Ophthalmol Strabismus* 34(3):190–192, 1997.

CHAPTER 6

RETINOPATHY OF PREMATURITY

TERRI L. YOUNG and DAVID B. SCHAFFER

DEFINITION OF TERMS

Retinopathy of prematurity (ROP) was first called *retrolental fibroplasia* (RLF) and described in the 1940s. It is associated with the use of excessive supplemental oxygen in neonatology practice to save premature infants. Despite more judicious use of oxygen in modern practice, ROP is now known to be a multifactorial disease and continues to be a potentially serious cause of ocular morbidity due to efforts to save ever-more-immature infants. In the Multicenter Trial of Cryotherapy for Retinopathy of Prematurity (CRYO-ROP) study, 65.8% of infants weighing less than 1251 g at birth showed evidence of some form of ROP, 16.5% had stage 3 disease, and 2.1% had unfavorable outcomes of macular folds or retinal detachments.

ROP is initially characterized by a fibroglial demarcation between vascularized posterior retina and avascular peripheral retina. More advanced stages exhibit abnormal neovascularization at this junction. With progressive vascular incompetence of the retinal vessels, a finding known as "plus" disease develops. Left untreated, the more advanced stages of the disease could lead to extensive fibrovascular proliferation, retinal traction, and retinal detachment, with subsequent severe visual loss (see Figs. 6-2 through 6-8).

DIFFERENTIAL DIAGNOSIS

1. Familial exudative vitreoretinopathy (FEVR) is characterized by peripheral vascular anomalies or absent vascularization of the retina. Ophthalmologic features are similar to those seen in ROP; systemic clinical features are normal (i.e., no prematurity and a normal birth history). Clinical manifestation can be extremely variable, ranging from peripheral vitreous strands to retinal folds and traction. Severe cases have both retinal detachment and phthisis bulbi. In the majority of patients, inheritance is autosomal dominant with high penetrance and variable expression. A gene for this form has been mapped to chromosome 11q13–q23. A few families with X-linked recessive inheritance have also been reported, with mapped loci at chromosomes Xq21.3 and Xp11.4.

2. Norrie's disease (ND) is an X-linked recessive disorder characterized by bilateral retinal dysplasia and accompanied by progressive hearing loss and central nervous system dysfunction in at least one-third of patients. Within the eye, neuronal retinal degenerative changes, retinal detachment, microphthalmia, cataract, corneal opacities, and persistent hyperplastic primary vitreous (PHPV) can be present. Norrin, the gene for ND, maps to chromosome Xp11.4.

3. X-linked primary retinal dysplasia is a peripheral retinopathy with macular fold, often accompanied with mental retardation and/or hearing loss.

4. Thrombophillic disorder or "compound heterozygous deficiency S" has vitreoretinal findings similar to severe ROP and has been described in neonatal siblings with thrombophilia.

5. Persistent hyperplastic primary vitreous (PHPV)

6. Ocular Toxocariasis

7. Coats' disease

8. Myopic degeneration

WORKUP

1. Gestational age, birth weight, and neonatal course are the leading clinical predictors of ROP, which occurs more commonly in the

smaller, sicker premature infants. The most serious stages of ROP occur in infants with birth weights less than 1000 g.

2. Routine surveillance with periodic dilated fundus examinations as per the recommendations of the CRYO-ROP Study Group using the International Classification of Retinopathy of Prematurity (ICROP).

CLASSIFICATION

The ICROP was developed in the early 1980s as a consensus document by an international group of ophthalmologists from eleven countries with particular interest in this disorder. Recorded findings of acute-phase ROP using the ICROP system have become standard in most nurseries. It consists of four basic elements: zone, stage, extent, and the presence or absence of plus disease. Zones are created by dividing the retina into three concentric circles centered around the optic disc. This permits description of the anterior-posterior location of the retinopathy. Zone 1 is the most posterior and zone 3 is the most peripheral. Zone 1 is defined as the area within a circle centered on the disc and has a radius of twice the disc-foveal distance. Zone 2 extends from the edge of zone 1 to a circle with a radius the distance from the disc to the nasal ora serrata. Zone 3 is the temporal crescent-shaped retinal area peripheral to zone 2 (Fig. 6-1). The extent of retinopathy along the circumference of the vascularized retina is described in terms of 30° sectors or clock hours of ROP. The term *plus disease* is used to designate the presence of engorged and tortuous vessels of the posterior pole (Fig. 6-2) and is sometimes also seen in the iris vasculature (Fig. 6-3). Both indicate a more advanced and aggressive form of retinopathy.

Severity of acute-phase retinopathy at the junction between the avascular and vascular peripheral retina is described by the stage of ROP. Five stages of retinopathy from the early vascular changes to partial or total retinal detachment are described. Stage 1 ROP is described as a demarcation line, which is a thin, flat, white line between vascularized and gray avascular retina (Fig. 6-4). Stage 2 ROP consists of a ridge or an elevation and thickening of the retina in the region of the demarcation line (Fig. 6-5). In stage 3 ROP, fibrovascular proliferation from the region of the ridge extends into the vitreous, with neovascularization at the ridge (Fig. 6-6). Stage 4 ROP is subdivided into two categories: Stage 4A, a partial retinal detachment sparing the foveal region, and stage 4B, in which the partial detachment involves the foveal region (Fig. 6-7). In stage 5 ROP, a total retinal detachment is present with a funnel appearance, and the funnel may be open or closed anteriorly and/or posteriorly (Fig. 6-8).

SCREENING FOR ROP

A 1996 joint statement from the American Academy of Pediatrics, the American Association for Pediatric Ophthalmology and Strabismus, and the American Academy of Ophthalmology suggested the following guidelines for screening examinations for ROP: infants with birth weights ≤ 1500 g or gestational age ≤ 28 weeks should be screened. In addition, higher-birth-weight infants who had an unstable clinical course and were therefore at high risk for ROP as determined by the neonatologist should also be examined. An experienced ophthalmologist familiar with the ICROP who routinely examines infants should perform the screening examinations using indirect ophthalmoscopy and scleral depression. Initial examinations should begin when the infant is 4 to 6 weeks after birth or in the 31- to 33-week postconceptional age window. Subsequent examinations are determined by the findings at the initial examination. They should generally occur every 1 to 2 weeks and vary depending on the location and severity of retinopathy, or the extent of retinal vascularization when no ROP is observed.

Mutations of the ND gene have been reported in patients with advanced ROP. This suggests that mutations in the ND gene may be responsible for advanced ROP in a subset of predisposed infants. An ROP-like presentation has been noted in infants with thrombophilic disorders. Future directions in prevention and diagnosis may include screening for mutations in the ND gene, as well as factor V, prothrombin, antithrombin III, protein C, protein S, cystathione β-synthetase, and methylenetetrahydrofolate reductase genes.

TREATMENTS

Treatment modalities during pregnancy that lead to fewer premature deliveries would diminish the prevalence of ROP. It is possible that combination therapies, both medical and surgical, may yield the best long-term results. Furthermore, providing aggressive supportive care for sepsis, hypoxia, hyperoxia, and acute illness in premature infants will no doubt affect the incidence and severity of ROP.

The national CRYO-ROP study was designed to determine the efficacy of cryotherapy in preventing progression to blindness in severe ROP. Transscleral cryotherapy was applied to the avascular retina of randomly selected eyes of 291 infants who had "threshold" ROP, defined as at least five contiguous or eight cumulative clock hours of stage 3 ROP in zone 1 or 2 in the presence of plus disease (Fig. 6-9). The 1988 and 1990 reports of the results showed that posterior retinal detachment, retinal fold involving the macula, or retrolental tissue (Fig. 6-10) obscuring the posterior pole was significantly less common in eyes that had undergone cryotherapy, compared to eyes with threshold ROP which remained untreated (31.1% vs. 51.4%, $p < 0.000010$).

The current recommendations for treatment of threshold disease suggest cryotherapy or, now more commonly, laser ablation to the avascular retina within 48 to 72 hours of threshold diagnosis. Either technique may be performed under local or general anesthesia, and both are effective in preventing progression of disease in most, but not all, cases. Despite timely intervention at threshold ROP, retinal detachments still occur in eyes of infants. Scleral buckling procedures may be effective in some detachments, although vitrectomy procedures may be required in more extensive detachments. In these eyes, outlook for functional vision is poor and the prognosis is guarded.

CONCLUSIONS

Despite advances in our understanding and management of ROP, it remains a leading cause of blindness in children in the United States. Vigilant surveillance and timely treatment remain our best defenses against this disorder.

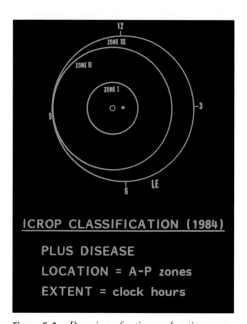

Figure 6-1 *Drawing of retina and optic nerve used by the International Classification of Retinopathy of Prematurity (ICROP) system for description standardization. Since retinal angiogenesis begins at the optic disc and spreads equally in both the temporal and nasal directions, it is the center of zones 1 and 2. The remaining temporal crescent of retina is the last to vascularize and is zone 3.*

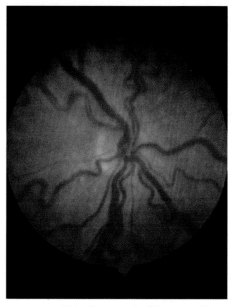

Figure 6-2 *This photograph of the optic disc and posterior retina depicts typical plus disease with arterial and venous tortuosity and engorgement of all four quadrants of the posterior retinal vasculature.*

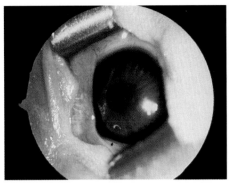

Figure 6-3 *This photograph of the cornea and iris shows anterior plus disease with iris vasculature engorgement and poor pupillary dilation.*

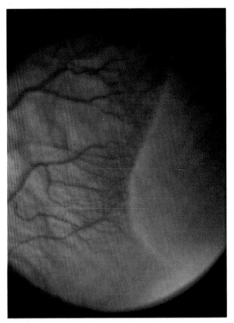

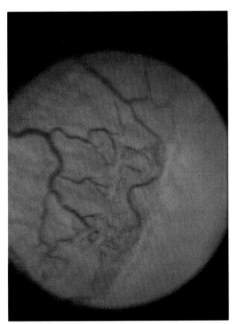

Figure 6-4 *This photograph of the peripheral retina shows stage 1 ROP with a demarcation line between vascularized and avascular retina within the plane of the retina.*

Figure 6-5 *This photograph of the peripheral retina shows stage 2 ROP with a demarcation ridge (height and width) between vascular and avascular retina. There are formations of fibroglial tissue posterior to the ridge called "popcorns."*

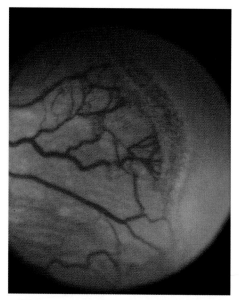

Figure 6-6 *This photograph of the peripheral retina shows stage 3 ROP with a thickened ridge and neovascular tissue emanating from the ridge into the vitreous. These abnormal blood vessels will bleed and stimulate the production of fibrovascular proliferation in the vitreous, leading to scarring and tractional retinal detachment. (Courtesy of John T. Flynn, M.D., Bascom Palmer Eye Institute.)*

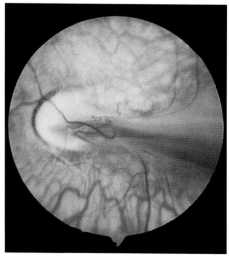

Figure 6-7 *This photograph of the posterior retina shows stage 4B ROP with a focal retinal detachment involving the macula. This outcome of ROP results in severe visual loss.*

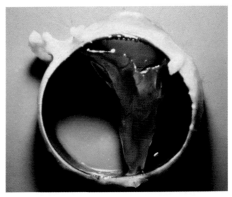

Figure 6-8 *This photograph of a sectioned, enucleated globe shows stage 5 ROP with a complete funnel retinal detachment.*

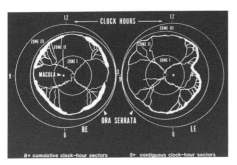

Figure 6-9 *Drawing of retina and optic nerve used by the ICROP system for description standardization. This drawing depicts the clinical condition of "threshold" ROP, which is the point at which the criteria for treatment have been met. These are five contiguous or eight cumulative clock hours of stage 3 in zone 2 with* plus disease.

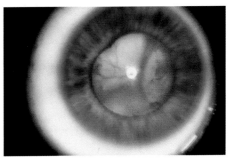

Figure 6-10 *This photograph of the cornea and iris shows a retrolental fibroproliferative membrane (old nomenclature, RLF) adherent to the posterior aspect of the lens with stage 5 ROP. (Courtesy of William Tasman, M.D., Wills Eye Hospital.)*

SELECTED REFERENCES

Chen Z-Y et al: A mutation in the Norrie disease gene (NDP) associated with X-linked familial exudative vitreoretinopathy. *Nat Genet* 5:180–183, 1993.

Cryotherapy for Retinopathy of Prematurity Cooperative Group: Natural history of retinopathy of prematurity (ROP): the natural outcome of premature birth and retinopathy: status at one year. *Arch Ophthalmol* 12:903–912, 1994.

The Cryotherapy for ROP Cooperative Group: Multicenter trial of cryotherapy for ROP: one year outcome—structure and function. *Arch Ophthalmol* 108:1408–1416, 1990.

Fullwood P et al: X-linked exudative vitreoretinopathy: clinical features and genetic linkage analysis. *Br J Ophthalmol* 77:168–170, 1993.

ICROP Committee for Classification of Late Stages of ROP: An international classification of retinopathy of prematurity: II. The classification of retinal detachment. *Arch Ophthalmol* 105:906–912, 1987.

ICROP Committee: International classification of retinopathy of prematurity. *Arch Ophthalmol* 102:1130–1134, 1984.

Mintz-Hittner H et al: Peripheral retinopathy in offspring of carriers of Norrie disease gene mutations. *Ophthalmology* 103:2128–2134, 1996.

Mintz-Hittner HA et al: Vitreoretinal findings similar to retinopathy of prematurity in infants with compound heterozygous protein S deficiency. *Ophthalmology* 106:1525–1530, 1999.

Palmer EA et al for the Cryotherapy for ROP Cooperative Group: Incidence and early course of retinopathy of prematurity. *Ophthalmology* 98:1628–1640, 1991.

Phelps DL: Retinopathy of prematurity: an estimate of vision loss in the United States— 1979. *Pediatrics* 67:924–926, 1981.

Pierce EA, Mukai S: Controversies in the management of retinopathy of prematurity. *Int Ophthalmol Clin* 34:121–148, 1994.

Schaffer DB et al for the Cryotherapy for ROP Cooperative Group: Prognostic factors in the natural course of ROP. *Ophthalmology* 100:230–237, 1993.

Shastry BS et al: Linkage and candidate gene analysis of X-linked familial exudative vitreoretinopathy. *Genomics* 27:341–344, 1995.

Shastry BS et al: Identification of missense mutations in the Norrie disease gene associated with advanced retinopathy of prematurity. *Arch Opthalmol* 115:651–655, 1997.

Shastry BS, Hejtmancik JF, Trese MT: Identification of novel missense mutations in the Norrie disease gene associated with one X-linked and four sporadic cases of familial exudative vitreoretinopathy. *Hum Mutat* 9:396–401, 1997.

PART II

OPHTHALMIC DISEASE IN INFANTS

CHAPTER 7

STRABISMUS IN INFANCY

JOHN M. AVALLONE

DEFINITIONS OF TERMS

The word *strabismus* has its origin from the Greek *strabos,* which means "crooked" or to "squint." Strabismus is any condition where the eyes are misaligned. The incidence of strabismus in the pediatric population is approximately 4%. Left untreated, the misalignment will persist into adulthood. The etiology of strabismus remains obscure, but there is some genetic component. In children who have strabismus, studies have shown that the incidence of strabismus in the family ranges from 17.6% to 45.6%. In one study of 38,000 children between the ages of 1 and 2.5 years, the incidence of strabismus was 1.3%. Esotropia represented 72%, exotropia accounted for 23%, and the remainder was vertical strabismus at 4.6%.

Strabismus can be divided into two main types: comitant and noncomitant. Comitant means that the eye misalignment is the same in all gaze positions, and noncomitant means that the misalignment is different in various gaze positions. That division helps define etiology, because comitant deviations imply cortical origin (supranuclear) and noncomitant deviations imply an origin at, or distal to, the midbrain (infranuclear). Strabismus can be further subdivided into horizontal and vertical misalignments. The horizontal misalignments consist of convergent (esotropia) and divergent (exotropia) types. Vertical misalignments are called hypertropias, based on the elevated eye.

Over 50% of children with strabismus will have amblyopia (loss of vision in one of the two eyes), emphasizing the need for early recognition and treatment of this disorder. The appropriate referral for pediatric patients with strabismus falls largely on the primary care community and vision screening programs in schools and neighborhoods. Strabismus is a sig-

nificant structural abnormality of the face. Over 50% of children with strabismus report being ridiculed about their eye alignment by their peers. Strabismus is seen with higher frequency in premature children and those with craniofacial disorders and cerebral palsy, but the majority of patients are neurologically normal.

Before 3 months of age a normal child's eye alignment may be esotropic or exotropic. A large portion (33% to 80%) of normal newborn children shows a tendency toward divergent (exotropic) deviations. This pattern moves toward no deviation between 2 and 4 months of age, with a significant decrease in prevalence of an ocular deviation at this time. Beyond 6 months of age there should be no eye misalignment in the normal child.

DIAGNOSIS

The simplest way to assess eye alignment in the office is to examine the corneal light reflexes of a patient looking at a penlight. If one eye is looking at the light and one eye is misaligned, then the light reflex will be displaced off the pupil in the nonfixing eye. If it is a convergent misalignment, then the light reflex will be displaced temporally on the nonfixing eye. Conversely, a divergent misalignment will show a nasally displaced light reflex on the nonfixing eye. A vertical misalignment will show the light reflex deflected up or down on the nonfixing eye. An eye-care practitioner accomplishes the definitive diagnosis after obtaining a history and physical examination. The most important part of the physical examination is the cover-uncover and alternate cover tests. The eye-care practitioner performs these tests to diagnose and quantitate the strabismus. Occasionally, radiographic imaging and laboratory testing are needed to aid in the diagnosis of strabismus type, particularly those associated with systemic and neurologic disease.

DIFFERENTIAL DIAGNOSIS

The differential diagnosis for esotropia in infancy is shown in Table 7-1. A common condition is "congenital esotropia." The incidence is approximately 1% of infants. This condition has also been called *essential infantile esotropia* or the *infantile esotropia complex or syndrome.* This "syndrome" is apparent by 6 months of age. It is characterized by onset in the first 6 months of life, a large-angle esotropic deviation, stable amount of eye crossing, lack of improvement with antiaccommodative therapy (glasses), and normal neurologic status. These patients will likely develop a vertical deviation to accompany their horizontal deviation over time, and nystagmus may be apparent as well. This constellation of findings forms the core of the syndrome. The horizontal deviation will be the most discernible component of the complex. Most of these children will alternate fixation between their two eyes. Of these children, 40% will develop amblyopia secondary to their esotropia because of some fixation preference. The treatment is surgical, and about half will require glasses after surgery to help maintain their eye alignment.

Table 7-1   DIFFERENTIAL DIAGNOSIS OF CONVERGENT STRABISMUS IN THE INFANT

1. Pseudoesotropia (Fig. 7-1)
2. Congenital esotropia "syndrome" (Figs. 7-7 and 7-8)
3. Duane retraction syndrome (a developmental absence of the sixth cranial nerve)
4. Accommodative esotropia (a form of esotropia associated with farsightedness and more commonly seen from 2 to 3 years of age)
5. Sensory deprivation esotropia (seen in children with monocular lesions that reduce vision in one eye, e.g., cataract, ptosis, intraocular mass, corneal scarring) (Figs. 7-13 and 7-14)
6. Cranial nerve VI palsy (idiopathic, traumatic, associated with raised intracranial pressure, and postinfectious)
7. Esotropia with central nervous system anomalies (cerebral palsy, hydrocephalus, Down's syndrome, etc.)

The differential diagnosis of esotropia also includes pseudoesotropia, a condition that may mimic esotropia because of the epicanthal skin folds on the child's nose. As the midface develops, these skin folds will diminish and the eyes will appear more normal.

Exotropia may develop in the first 6 months of life as well. Congenital exotropia is a very uncommon condition that presents early in life with a large-angle deviation. Exotropia in infancy is often associated with neurologic disease and developmental delays. These children will suffer some of the same sensory difficulties as children with congenital esotropia (Fig. 7-15).

Vertical misalignment may also be evident in this age group and may present as an abnormal head position as the child gains head and neck control (Figs. 7-11, 7-12, 7-16).

WORKUP

1. History—Complete ophthalmic and family history. Special attention to pregnancy, labor, delivery, and general growth and development. Family history of childhood eye problems, strabismus, patching, or glasses.
2. Ophthalmic examination—Vision assessment, pupils, external eye and motility examination, dilated intraocular exam, and refraction.
3. Radiographic imaging, laboratory and special testing—CT scan, MRI, serology (as indicated by history), and visual evoked responses, electroretinography and ocular motility recordings as indicated by ophthalmic exam.

TREATMENT GENERALITIES

1. Medical—The following are those general medical treatments available to the eye-care practitioner; the use and indications for each are beyond the scope of this atlas. The reader is referred to multiple excellent texts for further clarification. Common treatments include spectacles, occlusion (if amblyopia is present), miotic eye drops, prism glasses, and orthoptics (visual training) and botulinum toxin (Botox, Oculinum) injection into the extraocular muscles.
2. Surgical—The general indication for surgery includes the failure of medical treatment to result in improved binocular

cooperation. Surgery involves either "weakening" (recessing) or "strengthening" (resecting) an extraocular muscle. The purpose of these procedures is to align the eyes in a more favorable position for the brain to use them together. This is effective in 60% to 90% of patients, depending on the diagnosis.

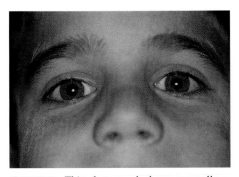

Figure 7-1 *This photograph shows normally centered corneal reflexes in both eyes.*

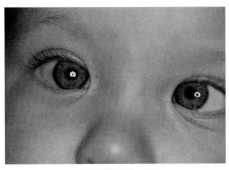

Figure 7-2 *This photograph shows a temporally displaced corneal reflex in the nonfixing left eye of a child with esotropia.*

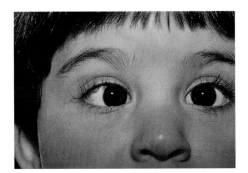

Figure 7-3 *This photograph shows a temporally displaced corneal reflex in the nonfixing right eye of a child with esotropia.*

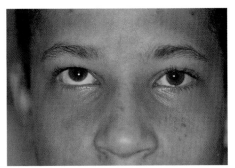

Figure 7-4 *This photograph shows an inferiorly displaced corneal reflex in the nonfixing right eye of a child with a right hypertropia.*

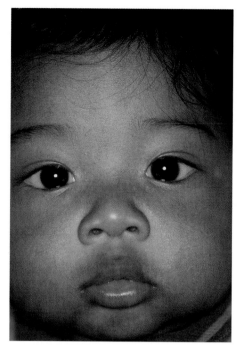

Figure 7-5 *This photograph shows normally centered corneal reflexes in both eyes in a child with large epicanthal eyelid folds called* pseudostrabismus.

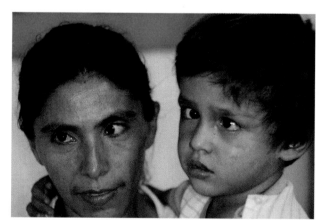

Figure 7-6 *This photograph shows a mother and child with untreated, basic childhood esotropia.*

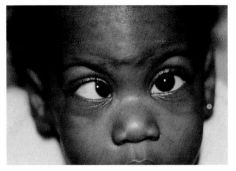 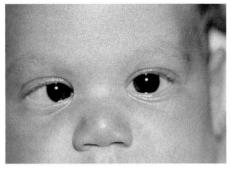

Figures 7-7 and 7-8 *These photographs show children with the infantile esotropia syndrome (congenital esotropia). This syndrome consists of a large-angle esotropia (Figs. 7-7 and 7-8) occurring in the first few months of life, nystagmus, alternating fixation, 40% incidence of amblyopia, overaction of the inferior oblique muscles, low levels of farsightedness, the dissociated strabismus complex (upward and outward drifting of one eye), and often a positive family history of strabismus or amblyopia.*

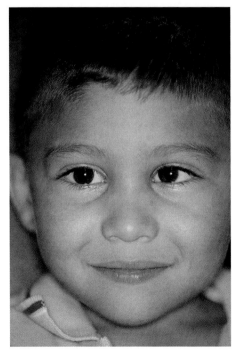 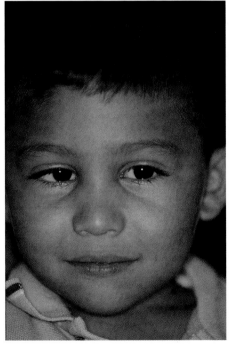

Figures 7-9 and 7-10 *These photographs show a child with esotropia and alternate fixation. Figure 7-9 shows the right eye fixing and the left crossed, and Fig. 7-10 shows spontaneous switching to the left eye while the right eye is now crossed.*

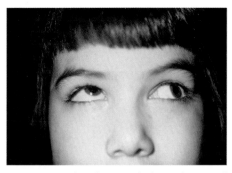

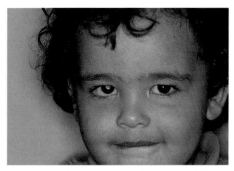

Figure 7-11   *This photograph shows the typical appearance, in the right eye, of the vertical deviation, "overaction of the inferior oblique." This deviation commonly accompanies both esotropic and exotropic childhood horizontal deviations.*

Figure 7-12   *This photograph shows a child with a sensory esotropia and a "white" reflex in the crossed right eye due to an intraocular retinoblastoma of that eye.*

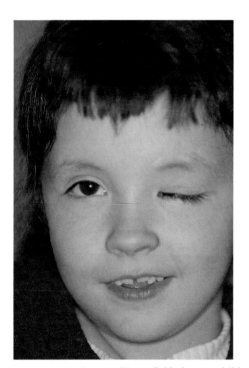

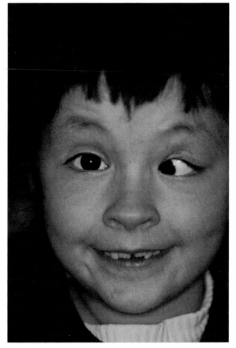

Figures 7-13 and 7-14   *Figure 7-13 shows a child with almost complete congenital ptosis of the left eye and almost no levator muscle function. She has a coincidental severe sensory esotropia illustrated by the left eye deviation shown in Fig. 7-14 after the left upper has been surgically elevated.*

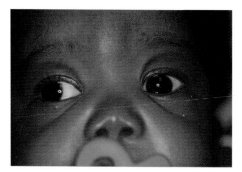

Figure 7-15 *This photograph shows a child with infantile exotropia and the right eye deviating temporally. This is important for the clinician to recognize, because this ocular deviation in infancy is more often associated with other central nervous system abnormalities and/or developmental delays.*

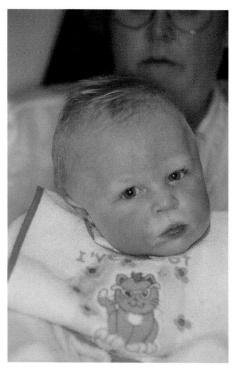

Figure 7-16 *This photograph shows a child with an anomalous head posture due to a congenital superior oblique paresis on the left side. This is characterized by an early-onset head tilt and vertical strabismus. The strabismus is classically a hypertropia with the head straight and is worse on head tilt toward the affected eye and decreased on head tilt toward the unaffected eye. Although damage to the fourth cranial nerve can cause this, most of these cases are due to developmental anomalies of the superior oblique tendon, leading to poor function.*

SELECTED REFERENCES

Cibis GW: Comitant strabismus. *Curr Opin Ophthalmol* 9(5):15–19, 1998.

de Farber JT, Kingma-Wilschut C, Grootendorst R: Comitant strabismus. *Curr Opin Ophthalmol* 10(5):305–309, 1999.

Helveston EM: The value of strabismus surgery. *Ophthalmic Surg* 21(5):311–317, 1990.

Hunter DG, Ellis FJ: Prevalence of systemic and ocular disease in infantile exotropia: comparison with infantile esotropia. *Ophthalmology* 106(10):1951–1956, 1999.

LaRoche GR: Paralytic strabismus. *Curr Opin Ophthalmol* 10(5):310–313, 1999.

Nelson LB et al: Congenital esotropia. *Surv Ophthalmol* 31(6):363–383, 1987.

Parks MM: Congenital esotropia vs infantile esotropia. *Graefes Arch Clin Exp Ophthalmol* 226(2):106–107, 1988.

Paul TO, Hardage LK: The heritability of strabismus. *Ophthalmic Genet* 15(1):1–18, 1994.

Raab EL: The strabismus patient: an outline of examination and treatment. *Sight Sav Rev* 47(4):157–165, 1977.

Wilson ME, Hutchinson AK, Saunders RA: Outcomes from surgical treatment for dissociated horizontal deviation. *J Pediatr Ophthalmol Strabismus* 4(2):94–101, 2000.

CHAPTER 8

SYSTEMIC GENETIC CRANIOFACIAL SYNDROMES WITH OPHTHALMIC INVOLVEMENT

RICHARD W. HERTLE and JILL A. FOSTER

DEFINITIONS OF TERMS

Ocular genetic disorders affect all parts of the visual system. Almost every autosome and the X chromosome have genes that have been implicated in causing an ocular condition. Specific areas in which genetic abnormalities have been discovered include myopia; lids and adnexa; anterior segment and lens; tumors of the eye, orbit, and lids; craniofacial anomalies; glaucoma; retinal degenerations and dystrophies; optic neuropathies; brain deformities; and strabismus and eye-movement disorders.

DIFFERENTIAL DIAGNOSIS

All children with multiple malformations should have chromosomal analysis. Chromosomal anomalies are distinguished from single-gene defects in that they involve a gross structural change (extra or absent material) of the chromosome. These patients benefit from a full clinical and molecular genetics analysis. This is used to provide information regarding carrier detection, presymptomatic evaluation, and prenatal diagnosis and counseling (Figs. 8-1 to 8-12).

CHROMOSOMAL ABNORMALITIES INVOLVING THE VISUAL SYSTEM

1. Trisomy 13, 15, and 18
2. Trisomy 21 (Down syndrome)
3. Triploidy
4. "Cat's-eye" syndrome (tetrasomy of 22q11)
5. 11p13 deletion (aniridia, Wilm's tumor)
6. 4p16 Deletion (Wolf-Hirshhorn syndrome)
7. 45X/46XX (Turner's syndrome)
8. 5p– (cri-du-chat syndrome)

CRANIOFACIAL SYNDROMES

The craniofacial syndromes are a group of cranial vault and facial malformations affecting normal development and growth. They may be associated with systemic manifestations such as limb, spine, and central nervous system abnormalities. They are divided into clefting syndromes and synostotic (premature closure of the cranial sutures) syndromes. In recent years many of these syndromes have had their underlying genetic defect discovered. Of particular interest is the finding of abnormalities of the fibroblast growth factor receptor gene defect in many forms of synostoses. The visual system and ocular structures are commonly affected in this group of diseases (Figs. 8-13 to 8-30). The major ophthalmic consequences include orbital dystopia, hypertelorism, telecanthus, exorbitism, lid colobomas, ptosis, canthal dystopia, globe exposure and keratitis, strabismus, amblyopia, high refractive errors, cataracts, glaucoma, and retinal and optic nerve dysplasia. The following is a brief classification.

Clefting Syndromes

1. Tessier clefts 0 to 10 (including cleft lip and palate)
2. Bifacial and hemifacial microsomia

3. Oculoaurovertebral dysplasia (e.g., Goldenhar's syndrome)
4. Treacher Collins syndrome

Craniosynostoses

1. Crouzon's syndrome
2. Apert's syndrome
3. Pfeiffer syndrome
4. Saethre-Chotzen syndrome
5. Carpenter's syndrome
6. Kleeblattschadel's anomaly

WORKUP

1. Full family and parental history
2. Complete ophthalmic examination.
3. Multiple specialty consultations, e.g., pediatrics, genetics, craniofacial/plastic reconstructive surgery, neurosurgery, otolaryngology, speech and feeding therapy, and psychiatry/social work.

OPHTHALMIC CONSEQUENCES

1. Optic nerve disease (dysplasia, hypoplasia, compressive neuropathy)
2. Orbital disease (exorbitism, hypertelorism, dystopia, hypoplasia)

3. Lid and adnexal disease (ptosis, malpositions, nasolacrimal duct obstruction)
4. Globe disorders (exposure keratitis, cataracts, glaucoma, colobomas)
5. Strabismus, nystagmus, and amblyopia
6. High refractive errors

TREATMENT

1. These patients require multiple ophthalmic medical and surgical treatments throughout the course of their childhood. These treatments are often coordinated with other "team" members caring for the patients and their families.
2. The ophthalmologist must be vigilant in the diagnosis and treatment of amblyopia, because this is the leading cause of visual loss in this patient population.

CONCLUSIONS

Although the group of genetic and craniofacial diseases requiring ophthalmic consultation is rare, the total number is so large that each eye-care professional involved with the pediatric population will be asked to examine and/or care for these patients.

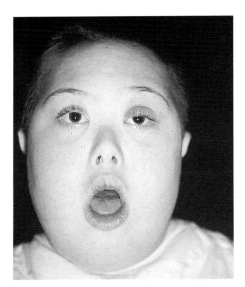
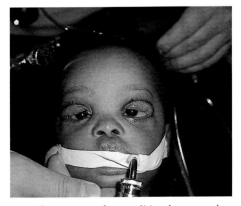

Figures 8-1 and 8-2 *Trisomy 21, one of the most common chromosome abnormalities, has a number of ocular findings, including bilateral epicanthal folds and oblique and shortened palpebral fissures (Fig. 8-1). Patients may also have lid malpositions such as ptosis (Fig. 8-1) or ectropion (Fig. 8-2). Other associated features may include iris "Brushfield" spots, cataracts, glaucoma, nystagmus, strabismus, high refractive errors, amblyopia, and optic nerve dysplasia.*

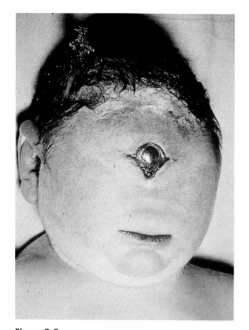

Figure 8-3

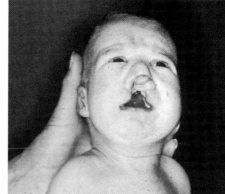

Figure 8-4

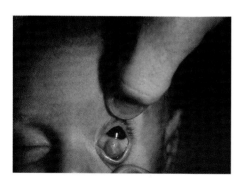

Figure 8-5

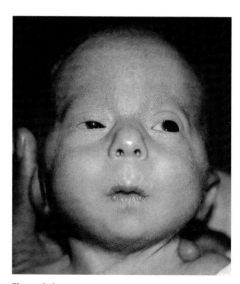

Figure 8-6

Figures 8-3 to 8-6   *Trisomy 18 and 13 are, respectively, the second and third most common autosomal trisomies. Systemic features of trisomy 13 include retardation, spina bifida, polydactyly, facial clefting, holoprosencephaly, hemangiomas, and internal organ defects. Ocular features can include cyclopia (Fig. 8-3), microcephaly, microphthalmos (Fig. 8-4), colobomas with or without associated cyst (Fig. 8-5), intraocular cartilage, and retinal dysplasia. Trisomy 18 is associated with early death due to heart disease or brainstem dysfunction. Ocular abnormalities include microphthalmos, cataract, cloudy corneas, colobomas, and also retinal dysplasia (Fig. 8-6).*

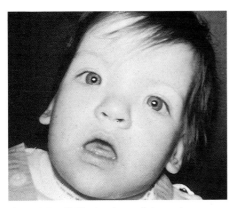

Figure 8-7 *Criduchat (cry-of-the-cat) syndrome is due to a partial deletion of chromosome 5; features include microcephaly, round face, low-set ears, hypotonia, facial clefting, catlike cry, and heart defects. Ocular features include hypertelorism, slanted palpebral fissures, epicanthus, strabismus, and optic atrophy.*

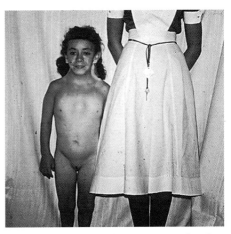

Figure 8-8 *Turner syndrome occurs in females with only one structural or functional X chromosome. This abnormality is characterized by short stature, webbing of the neck, and heart disease. Ocular findings consist of strabismus, refractive errors, ptosis, amblyopia, and red-green color deficiency.*

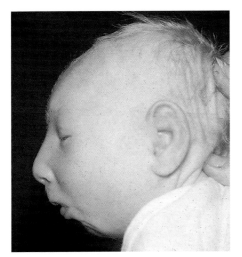

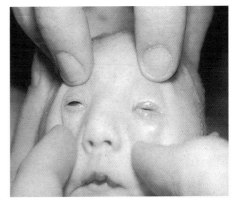

Figures 8-9 and 8-10 *In this condition there is an extra haploid set of chromosomes, e.g., 69 in triploidy and 92 in tetraploidy (Figs. 8-9 and 8-10). Although many of these patients are stillborn, some with mosaicism survive. Systemically many have brain malformations, spina bifida, flat midface with upturned nose, and syndactyly. Ocular features are common and include anophthalmia, microphthalmia, coloboma, retinal dysplasia, persistent primary vitreous, cataract, and glaucoma.*

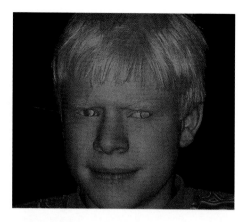

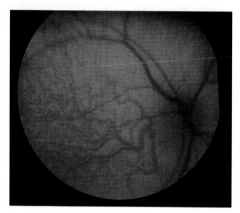

Figures 8-11 and 8-12 *Albinism is an inherited disease is due to abnormalities in the enzymatic pathway of tyrosine and is associated with deficient or absent pigment in the skin, hair, and eyes (Fig. 8-11). Ocular findings are present from birth and include abnormal decussation of the visual pathways within the brain; iris transillumination; nystagmus; strabismus; photophobia; and decreased vision due to foveal dysplasia, amblyopia, and high refractive errors. Figure 8-12 shows vessels through the retinal area where the foveal reflex would normally appear.*

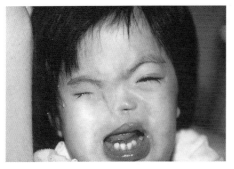

Figure 8-13

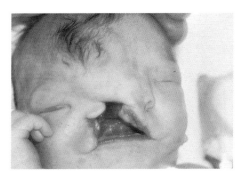

Figure 8-14

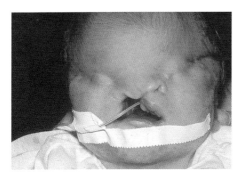

Figure 8-15

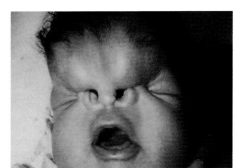

Figure 8-16

Figures 8-13 to 8-20 *Clefting syndromes include "Tessier" facial clefts that are due to interrupted fusion of embryonic facial processes and grooves. The most common classic clefts are depicted in Figs. 8-13 to 8-15. A severe form of midline facial cleft involving the intracranial structures is frontonasal dysplasia, depicted in Fig. 8-16. Other common clefting syndromes include bifacial and/or hemifacial microsomia (Figs. 8-17 and 8-18) with or without associated ear and eye deformities. These anomalies present in a broad spectrum of clinical conditions as part of the "oculo-auriculo-vertebral" syndromes, e.g., Goldenhar's syndrome and Treacher Collins syndrome (Figs. 8-19 and 8-20).*

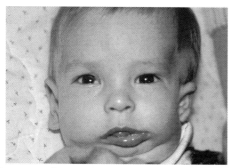

Figure 8-17

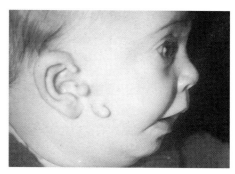

Figure 8-18

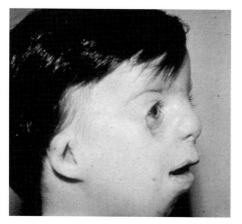

Figure 8-19

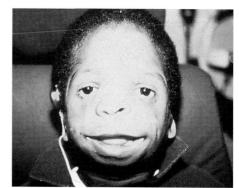

Figure 8-20

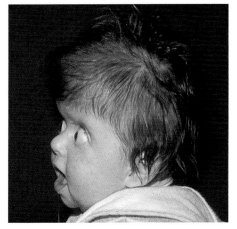

Figure 8-21

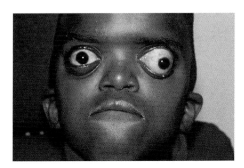

Figure 8-22

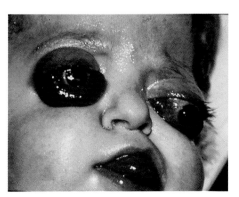

Figure 8-23

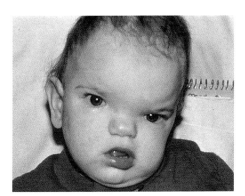

Figure 8-24

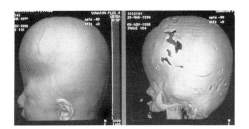

Figure 8-25

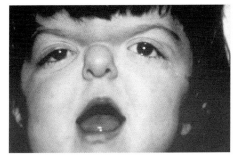

Figure 8-26

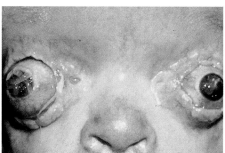

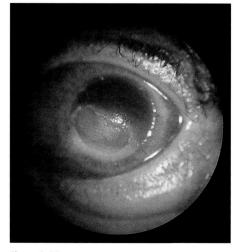

Figure 8-27

Figure 8-28

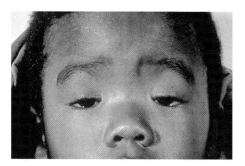

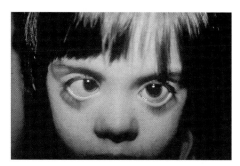

Figure 8-29

Figure 8-30

Figures 8-21 to 8-30 *Craniostenoses are a group of genetic syndromes due to premature closure of single or multiple cranial sutures with resultant deformities of the cranium and face. The most common suture involved is the coronal suture. Crouzon's syndrome is depicted in Figs. 8-21 to 8-23. Predominant findings of brachycephaly, exorbitism, and strabismus are depicted in these figures. Figure 8-24 illustrates the clinical appearance of "plagiocephaly" due to unilateral coronal suture synostoses. Figure 8-25 shows a three-dimensional CT scan reconstruction of this deformity. Figure 8-26 shows the typical midface crowding and down-slanting orbits associated with Apert's syndrome. This syndrome belongs to a large group of synostotic syndromes with associated syndactyly. Ophthalmic consequences of these syndromes include exorbitism with severe globe exposure (Figs. 8-27 and 8-28) and severe exposure keratitis. This is illustrated with fluorescein staining of the cornea in Fig. 8-28. Common lid malpositions include ptosis (Fig. 8-29) and ectropion of the lower lids (Fig. 8-30).*

SELECTED REFERENCES

Hertle RW: Ocular manifestations of genetic and developmental diseases. *Curr Opin Ophthalmol* 7:6; 72–79, 1996.

Hertle RW, Quinn G, Katowitz J: Ocular and adnexal findings in patients with facial microsomias. *Ophthalmology* 99:114–119, 1992.

Hertle RW, Ziylan S, Katowitz JA: Ophthalmic findings and visual prognosis in Treacher Collins' syndrome. *Br J Ophthalmol* 77:642–645, 1993.

Katowitz JA, Hertle RW, Quinn GE: Ophthalmic management of craniofacial anomalies. chap. 110 in W Tasman, E Jaeger, and A Biglan (eds). *Duanes Clinical Ophthalmology*. New York, Harper & Row, 1993.

McCarthy JG et al: Twenty-year experience with early surgery for craniosynostosis: II. The craniofacial synostosis syndromes and pansynostosis—results and unsolved problems. *Plast Reconstr Surg* 96(2):284–295; discussion 296–298, 1995.

Traboulsi EI: Ocular malformations and developmental genes (review). *J Am Assoc Pediatr Ophthalmol Strabismus* 2(6):317–323.

DEVELOPMENTAL VITREORETINAL DISEASE

ALBERT M. MAGUIRE

ALBINISM

DEFINITIONS OF TERMS

Albinism is a general term referring to an inherited condition of decreased pigmentation. When only the eye is clinically involved, the condition is referred to as *ocular albinism,* e.g., X-linked Nettleship-Falls disease. When pigmentary dilution is clinically apparent in both the skin and eyes, the condition is referred to as *oculocutaneous albinism,* e.g., autosomal recessive tyrosinase-positive albinism. Nystagmus and decreased vision are common to all forms of albinism due to incomplete development of the fovea (foveal hypoplasia). Patients with *albinoidism* have normal or minimally reduced vision and no nystagmus because they have normal foveal development. Chédiak-Higashi syndrome (albinism with susceptibility to infection) and Hermansky-Pudlak syndrome (albinism with bleeding diathesis) are two potentially lethal conditions associated with albinism that require medical consultation (Figs. 9-1–9-3).

DIFFERENTIAL DIAGNOSIS

1. Coloboma—Segmental chorioretinal aplasia, usually a normal fovea, no nystagmus
2. Choroideremia—X-linked family history, nyctalopia, tunnel vision, reduced to flat electroretinogram (ERG), no nystagmus
3. Gyrate atrophy—Nyctalopia, tunnel vision, reduced to flat ERG, hyperornithemia, no nystagmus

WORKUP

1. Complete physical examination
2. Medical history including bleeding and infection diathesis
3. Family history of inherited retinal conditions
4. History of prematurity, supplemental oxygen exposure, TORCH syndrome
5. Systemic review of systems for other anomalies, infection, trauma
6. Complete ophthalmic examination
7. Visual evoked response to assess asymmetry of afferent visual system projection and ERG (supranormal)

TREATMENTS

1. Associated strabismus, amblyopia, and nystagmus-induced head posture
2. Proper refraction and lens tinting

PERSISTENT HYPERPLASTIC PRIMARY VITREOUS

DEFINITIONS OF TERMS

Persistent hyperplastic primary vitreous (PHPV) is a congenital ocular malformation caused by incomplete regression of the primary vitreous. PHPV is typically a unilateral condition, but it may be bilateral when it occurs in association with systemic anomalies. It is present at birth in full-term infants without a history of supplemental oxygen exposure.

Depending on severity, PHPV will cause varying degrees of microphthalmia. Fibrovascular remnants of the vasa hyaloidea propria and/or primary vitreous can exist at any point along the axis between the optic disc and the posterior lens and ciliary body. Mittendorf's dot and Bergmeister's papilla are formes frustes of PHPV localized to the most anterior and posterior points of the primary vitreous. When fibroglial tissue and associated fibrovascular proliferation are pronounced, the effect on ocular growth and development is more severe. Anterior PHPV involves proliferation of tissue in the region of the ciliary body and retrolental space, Cloquet's canal. Anterior PHPV can manifest clinically with leukokoria, progressive cataract, glaucoma, and, in cases of severe ciliary body involvement, retinal detachment and cyclitic membrane or mass. Posterior PHPV occurs when fibrovascular proliferation in proximity to remnant hyaloid artery results in anatomic abnormalities of the optic disc and posterior pole. Papillary tractional elevation, tractional detachment of the retina, and macular pucker can be seen with posterior involvement. Most eyes will manifest varying degrees of anterior and posterior involvement with PHPV (Figs. 9-4–9-8).

DIFFERENTIAL DIAGNOSIS

1. Retinoblastoma—Average onset, 23 months; no vitreous membranes; calcium present
2. Posterior cataract—No persistent hyaloid vessel, no ciliary body membranes, usually bilateral with no microphthalmia
3. Infectious endophthalmitis—History of trauma or sepsis, acute pain with lid edema, severe purulent inflammation, positive cultures
4. Toxoplasmosis—Congenital with late reactivation, complaint of floaters, minimal vitreous membranes, no focal mass, positive serology for *Toxoplasma gondii* exposure
5. Pars planitis—Bilateral, mostly in males, peripheral mass with localized membranes
6. Retinopathy of prematurity—history of prematurity, neonatal onset, bilateral, no mass, no inflammation
7. Familial exudative vitreoretinopathy (FEVR)—Bilateral, family history, lipid exudation, no inflammation, no mass
8. Coats' disease—Mostly males, no inflammation, no membranes, severe lipid exudation

9. X-linked retinoschisis—Males only, family history, bilateral, foveal schisis, and other typical features

WORKUP

1. Family history of inherited retinal conditions
2. History of prematurity, supplemental oxygen exposure, TORCH syndrome
3. Systemic review of systems for other anomalies, infection, or trauma
4. Complete ophthalmic examination
5. Ultrasound examination for persistent hyaloid vessel, tractional detachment, calcium (absent), and biometry of *both* eyes to rule out subtle microphthalmia

TREATMENTS

PHPV is a surgically treated disease. Surgery is performed to treat glaucoma, to remove axial opacities (cataract), or to remove membranes causing tractional damage to the retina or ciliary body.
1. Vitrectomy or lensectomy with diathermy of the persistent hyaloid vessel (prevent intraocular hemorrhage).
2. Vitrectomy with membrane stripping for severe macular puckering (foveal development is often normal).
3. Pars plana is typically incompletely developed in PHPV, and therefore anterior entry sites or infusion is necessary to avoid retinal tears.

COATS' DISEASE

DEFINITIONS OF TERMS

First described in 1908 by Coats, Coats' disease is an exudative retinopathy caused by a congenital abnormality of the retinal vasculature. This condition occurs predominantly in males, and is almost always unilateral. The patient often presents with leukokoria, decreased vision, and/or strabismus. Coats' disease may cause profound, permanent visual impairment. The primary lesion is localized retinovascular telangiectasia with vascular incompetence. Leakage of serum elements from abnormal vessels leads to lipid deposition with subsequent subretinal fibrosis and to exudative retinal detachment. Clinically, lipid deposition tends to occur in the macular area, leading to central visual impairment. A milder form of Coats' disease occurring in adults is known as parafoveal telangiectasis type II (Figs. 9-9–9-12).

DIFFERENTIAL DIAGNOSIS

1. Familial exudative vitreoretinopathy (FEVR)—Bilateral, family history, lipid exudation, no inflammation, no mass
2. Retinoblastoma—average onset, 23 months; no vitreous membranes; calcium present
3. Infectious endophthalmitis—History of trauma or sepsis, acute pain with lid edema, severe purulent inflammation, positive cultures
4. Toxoplasmosis—Congenital with late reactivation, complaint of floaters, minimal vitreous membranes, no focal mass, positive serology for *T. gondii* exposure
5. Pars planitis—Bilateral, mostly in males, peripheral mass with localized membranes
6. Retinopathy of prematurity—History of prematurity, neonatal onset, bilateral, no mass, no inflammation
7. Persistent hyperplastic primary vitreous (PHPV)—Present at birth, microphthalmia, fibrovascular stalk from disc, no inflammation
8. X-linked retinoschisis—Males only, family history, bilateral, foveal schisis, and other typical features

WORKUP

1. Family history of inherited retinal conditions
2. History of prematurity, supplemental oxygen exposure, TORCH syndrome
3. Systemic review of systems for other anomalies, infection, trauma
4. Complete ophthalmic examination
5. Fluorescein angiography or angioscopy
6. Ultrasound examination to rule out preretinal membranes (absent), calcium (absent), and biometry of *both* eyes to rule out subtle microphthalmia (PHPV)

TREATMENTS

1. Severe cases—Cryotherapy
2. Mild cases—Laser photocoagulation

COLOBOMA

DEFINITIONS OF TERMS

Coloboma involving the retina and choroid is a developmental anomaly related to incomplete closure of the optic fissure. Coloboma may occur as a sporadic or inherited (autosomal dominant) trait, and is occasionally seen in association with systemic syndromes. Chorioretinal colobomas always involve tissue inferior to the optic nerve along the axis of the embryonic fissure. The macula is rarely contained in the coloboma, and therefore, in the absence of retinal detachment, central acuity is typically good. Clinically, chorioretinal colobomas appear as parabolic white areas of chorioretinal excavation sharply demarcated by normal-appearing retina. Extensive colobomas may give the appearance of leukokoria due to the large areas of sclera exposed by the chorioretinal defect. Occasionally, isolated rests of colobomatous tissue will reside along the embryonic fissure separated from the optic disc and peripheral retina. The central area within a coloboma contains gliotic tissue. Retinal breaks can occur along the edges of a coloboma, resulting in a rhegmatogenous retinal detachment (Figs. 9-13–9-15).

DIFFERENTIAL DIAGNOSIS

1. Toxoplasmosis—Congenital with late reactivation, complaint of floaters, minimal vitreous membranes, occurs anywhere in fundus including macula, no focal mass, positive serology for *T. gondii* exposure
2. Aicardi's syndrome—Early-onset infantile myoclonic seizures and flexor spasms, females, PHPV findings

WORKUP

1. Family history of inherited retinal conditions
2. History of prematurity, supplemental oxygen exposure, TORCH syndrome
3. Systemic review of systems for other anomalies, infection, trauma. Coloboma associations include CHARGE association, trisomy 13, Meckel syndrome, Warburg's syndrome, Aicardi's syndrome, and basal encephalocele

4. Complete ophthalmic examination
5. Complete ophthalmic examination of family members
6. Ultrasound examination for optic nerve and chorioretinal coloboma, and associated micropthalmia
7. Neuroimaging for midline developmental defects

TREATMENTS

1. Rhegmatogenous retinal detachment—Vitreous surgery with laser and intraocular gas or silicone oil tamponade for breaks along the border of the coloboma

OCULAR TOXOCARIASIS

DEFINITIONS OF TERMS

Ocular toxocariasis (OT) is an inflammatory condition of the retina and vitreous due to infestation of the posterior segment by the second-stage larvae of the roundworm *Toxocara canis.* Nematode endophthalmitis was first described in 1950 by Wilder. Nichols identified the etiologic agent as *T. canis* in 1956, the same infectious agent identified by Beaver in 1952 causing the systemic syndrome visceral larva migrans. OT patients present between 2 and 30 years of age, with average age of presentation of 8 years. OT accounted for 37% of retinal diagnoses in the pediatric age group in one ophthalmology practice. Epidemiologic studies have established that the risk of developing OT is related to pica behavior and close exposure to dogs. Ocular manifestations of OT include peripheral granuloma, posterior pole granuloma, and subacute or chronic endophthalmitis. Children typically present with unilateral decreased vision, strabismus, or leukokoria (Figs. 9-16 and 9-17).

DIFFERENTIAL DIAGNOSIS

1. Retinoblastoma—Average onset, 23 months; no vitreous membranes; calcium present
2. Infectious endophthalmitis—History of trauma or sepsis, acute pain with lid edema, severe purulent inflammation, positive cultures
3. Toxoplasmosis—Congenital with late reactivation, complaint of floaters, minimal vitreous membranes, no focal mass, positive serology for *T. gondii* exposure
4. Pars planitis—Bilateral, mostly in males, peripheral mass with localized membranes
5. Retinopathy of prematurity—History of prematurity, neonatal onset, bilateral, no mass, no inflammation
6. Persistent hyperplastic primary vitreous (PHPV)—Present at birth, microphthalmia, fibrovascular stalk from disc, no inflammation
7. Familial exudative vitreoretinopathy (FEVR)—Bilateral, family history, lipid exudation, no inflammation, no mass
8. Coats' disease—Mostly males, no inflammation, no membranes, severe lipid exudation
9. X-linked retinoschisis—Males only, family history, bilateral, foveal schisis, and other typical features

WORKUP

1. Family history of inherited retinal conditions
2. History of prematurity, supplemental oxygen exposure, TORCH syndrome
3. Behavior and social history of pica or close exposure to dogs, especially puppies
4. Systemic review of systems for other anomalies, infection, trauma
5. Complete ophthalmic examination
6. Complete blood count, intraocular fluid evaluation with differential (eosinophilia occasionally seen)
7. Serologic and intraocular fluid evaluation for *T. canis* antibodies
8. Ultrasound examination for persistent hyaloid vessel, tractional detachment, calcium (absent), and biometry of *both* eyes to rule out subtle microphthalmia (PHPV)

TREATMENTS

1. Anthelmintic drug therapy is not useful or indicated because the *T. canis* organism is not viable for long periods and does not migrate through the eye. Inflammation and membrane formation are the significant secondary complications of *T. canis* infection.
2. Vitreoretinal surgery for tractional complications

FAMILIAL EXUDATIVE VITREORETINOPATHY

DEFINITIONS OF TERMS

First described in 1969 by Criswick and Schepens, familial exudative vitreoretinopathy (FEVR) is an autosomal dominant disease affecting the peripheral retinal vasculature. This bilateral condition is seen in full-term children with normal developmental history. FEVR manifests with peripheral retinovascular nonperfusion, fibrovascular proliferation at the border of perfused and nonperfused retina, and marked retinovascular exudation. Traction from the fibrovascular mass can cause dragging of the disc, macular folds, and retinal detachment. Although highly penetrant, FEVR shows marked variability of expression, with some asymptomatic cases detectable only by fluorescein angiography. FEVR is rarely detected at birth, and usually shows progressive changes throughout childhood. The incidence of this disease is small, but is probably underestimated because clinicians overlook possible inheritance in asymptomatic individuals (Figs. 9-18–9-20).

DIFFERENTIAL DIAGNOSIS

1. Retinopathy of prematurity—History of prematurity, neonatal onset, bilateral, no mass, no inflammation
2. Persistent hyperplastic primary vitreous (PHPV)—Present at birth, microphthalmia, fibrovascular stalk from disc, no inflammation
3. Retinoblastoma—Average onset, 23 months; no vitreous membranes; calcium present
4. Infectious endophthalmitis—History of trauma or sepsis, acute pain with lid edema, severe purulent inflammation, positive cultures
5. Toxoplasmosis—Congenital with late reactivation, complaint of floaters, minimal vitreous membranes, no focal mass, positive serology for *T. gondii* exposure
6. Pars planitis—Bilateral, mostly in males, peripheral mass with localized membranes
7. Coats' disease—Mostly males, no inflammation, no membranes, severe lipid exudation

8. X-linked retinoschisis—Males only, family history, bilateral, foveal schisis, and other typical features

WORKUP

1. Family history of inherited retinal conditions
2. History of prematurity, supplemental oxygen exposure, TORCH syndrome
3. Systemic review of systems for other anomalies, infection, trauma
4. Complete ophthalmic examination
5. Complete ophthalmic examination of family members, including fluorescein angiography
6. Ultrasound examination for persistent hyaloid vessel, tractional detachment, calcium (absent), and biometry of *both* eyes to rule out subtle microphthalmia

TREATMENTS

1. Cryotherapy or laser photocoagulation to induce regression of neovascularization
2. Vitreoretinal surgery for tractional complications

LEBER'S CONGENITAL AMAUROSIS

DEFINITIONS OF TERMS

First described by Leber in 1869, Leber's congenital amaurosis (LCA) is a congenital retinal degeneration which presents in early infancy with profound visual impairment. In a Swedish population study, LCA was estimated to account for 10% of cases of congenital blindness, with an incidence of 3 per 100,000. Infants with LCA will show sluggish pupillary responses and searching nystagmus. ERG will demonstrate a severely attenuated or extinguished response. LCA has been classified as "uncomplicated" or "complicated" based on the presence of associated systemic findings. In uncomplicated LCA, high hyperopia is frequently seen and occasionally peculiar macular changes (e.g., pseudocoloboma) are present. The fundus will occasionally show pigment stippling early in the course of LCA, but frank pigmentary retinopathy is a late finding. In recent years, specific gene defects have been identified which may cause uncomplicated LCA. In complicated LCA, there are associated neurologic or other systemic abnormalities. This is no specific refractive error, and otherwise the ocular findings are similar to uncomplicated LCA (Fig. 9-21).

DIFFERENTIAL DIAGNOSIS

1. Early-onset or juvenile retinitis pigmentosa—No nystagmus, normal or myopic refraction, better central acuity than LCA
2. Coloboma—Inferior to optic nerve, rarely involves macula, parabolic white areas of chorioretinal excavation sharply demarcated by normal-appearing retina, retinal detachment
3. X-linked retinoschisis—Males only, family history, bilateral, foveal schisis, and other typical features

WORKUP

1. Family history of inherited retinal conditions
2. History of prematurity, supplemental oxygen exposure, TORCH syndrome
3. Systemic review of systems for other anomalies, infection, trauma
4. Complete ophthalmic examination
5. ERG

TREATMENTS

1. Supportive—As for low vision or blindness

AICARDI'S SYNDROME

DEFINITIONS OF TERMS

Aicardi's syndrome is an X-linked dominant disease that causes dysgenesis of the central nervous system and skeletal abnormalities. Aicardi's syndrome is seen almost exclusively in female infants because the genetic abnormality is lethal in XY males during embryonic development. Affected female infants are typically full-term and appear normal at birth. Infants present within a few weeks of age with myoclonic seizures and flexor spasms followed by severe psychomotor retardation. Ocular findings include pathognomonic chorioretinal "lacunae"—white, punched-out areas of atrophy involving the retinal pigment epithelium and choriocapillaris of 0.1 to 1.5 disc diameters

in size. These lacunae are often multiple and bilateral and usually occur in the inferior fundus. Other ocular findings may include developmental anomalies seen in PHPV, coloboma of the optic nerve or retina, optic nerve hypoplasia, and retinal detachment. Aicardi's syndrome is a lethal condition, with children rarely surviving past 2 years of age (Fig. 9-22).

DIFFERENTIAL DIAGNOSIS

1. Coloboma—Defects typically larger and more excavated than in Aicardi's syndrome, more severe alteration in architecture of overlying retina; coloboma may have association with basal encephalocele, has no seizure or spasm, occurs in males
2. Toxoplasmosis—Congenital with late reactivation, complaint of floaters, minimal vitreous membranes, no focal mass, positive serology for *T. gondii* exposure

WORKUP

1. Family history of inherited retinal conditions
2. History of prematurity, supplemental oxygen exposure, TORCH syndrome
3. Systemic review of systems for other anomalies, infection, trauma, myoclonic seizures, flexor spasm, hypertelorism, psychomotor retardation
4. Complete ophthalmic examination
5. Ultrasound examination for optic nerve and chorioretinal coloboma and associated microphthalmia
6. Neuroimaging to look for agenesis of corpus callosum, ventricular abnormalities; radiographs to look for fusion of thoracic vertebrae

TREATMENTS

1. None

X-LINKED JUVENILE RETINOSCHISIS

DEFINITIONS OF TERMS

This bilateral condition is seen in male children with normal birth and developmental history. Foveal schisis is a constant finding in X-linked retinoschisis, with petaloid cystic changes and radial striae resulting in moderate impairment in central visual acuity. Peripheral retinoschisis occurs in approximately 50% of patients, most commonly in the inferotemporal quadrants. The inner schisis layer (nerve fiber layer) can be highly elevated, with large holes and bridging retinal vessels. Vitreous hemorrhage can occur, with subsequent tractional changes. Rhegmatogenous retinal detachment rarely occurs when outer-layer breaks develop. X-linked retinoschisis is highly penetrant, but shows significant variability of expression, often with marked asymmetry between eyes. The clinical appearance of X-linked juvenile retinoschisis may show significant variation over time, with regression of large schisis cavities being quite common. The natural history of this disease is favorable, with mild progression occurring during childhood and little change after 20 years of age. Typically, patients maintain vision of 20/200 or better (Figs. 9-23–9-26).

DIFFERENTIAL DIAGNOSIS

1. FEVR—Peripheral retinovascular nonperfusion, fibrovascular proliferation, marked retinovascular exudation, no foveal schisis
2. Retinopathy of prematurity—History of prematurity, neonatal onset, bilateral, no mass, no inflammation
3. Persistent hyperplastic primary vitreous (PHPV)—Present at birth, microphthalmia, fibrovascular stalk from disc, no inflammation
4. Retinoblastoma—Average onset, 23 months; no vitreous membranes; calcium present
5. Infectious endophthalmitis—History of trauma or sepsis, acute pain with lid edema, severe purulent inflammation, positive cultures
6. Toxoplasmosis—Congenital with late reactivation, complaint of floaters, minimal vitreous membranes, no focal mass, positive serology for *T. gondii* exposure
7. Pars planitis—Bilateral, mostly in males, peripheral mass with localized membranes
8. Coats' disease—Mostly males, no inflammation, no membranes, severe lipid exudation

WORKUP

1. Family history of inherited retinal conditions

2. History of prematurity, administration of supplemental oxygen, TORCH syndrome
3. Systemic review of systems for other anomalies, infection, trauma
4. Complete ophthalmic examination
5. Complete ophthalmic examination of family members including fluorescein angiography (CME [cystoid macular edema] does *not* show fluorescein accumulation)
6. Ultrasound examination for persistent hyaloid vessel, tractional detachment, calcium (absent), and biometry of *both* eyes to rule out subtle microphthalmia

TREATMENTS

1. Rhegmatogenous retinal detachment (rare)—Vitreoretinal surgery
2. Vitreous hemorrhage—Observation

STARGARDT'S DISEASE

DEFINITIONS OF TERMS

Stargardt's disease is an early-onset inherited retinal degeneration that presents with reduced central visual acuity out of proportion to fundus changes. Often, subtle macular abnormalities are suspected of functional visual loss. With time macular changes become easily manifested, such as loss of foveal reflex, "beaten-bronze" foveal appearance, bull's-eye pigmentary changes, and appearance of pisciform yellow flecks surrounding the fovea. Central acuity declines rapidly within the first 10 to 20 years after presentation, with vision dropping to the 20/200 level. Other late signs include diffuse retinal pigment atrophy and/or bone spicule pigment migration. Abnormal accumulation of lipofuscin diffusely throughout the RPE accounts for blockage of choroidal fluorescence (choroidal silence) that is seen on fluorescein angiography in some patients (Figs. 9-27–9-29).

DIFFERENTIAL DIAGNOSIS

1. Toxoplasmosis—Congenital with late reactivation, complaint of floaters, minimal vitreous membranes, no focal mass, positive serology for *T. gondii* exposure
2. X-linked retinoschisis—Males only, family history, bilateral, foveal schisis, and other typical features

3. Coloboma—Inferior to optic nerve, rarely involves macula, parabolic white areas of chorioretinal excavation sharply demarcated by normal-appearing retina, occasionally retinal detachment
4. Leber's congenital amaurosis—Presents shortly after birth, sluggish pupillary responses, searching nystagmus, ERG severely attenuated or extinguished
5. Cone dystrophy—Early onset, diagnostic ERG with characteristic selective cone involvement, hemeralopia

WORKUP

1. Family history of inherited retinal conditions
2. History of prematurity, supplemental oxygen exposure, TORCH syndrome
3. Systemic review of systems for other anomalies, infection, trauma
4. Complete ophthalmic examination
5. Fluorescein angiography
6. DNA screening for ABCR mutations
7. Electrophysiology—May show normal or decreased ERG responses but no diagnostic pattern

TREATMENTS

1. Supportive—Low-vision rehabilitation

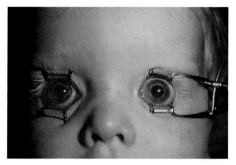 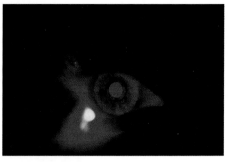

Figures 9-1 and 9-2 *The typical facial appearance (Fig. 9-1) and iris transillumination (Fig. 9-2) defects in a child with albinism.*

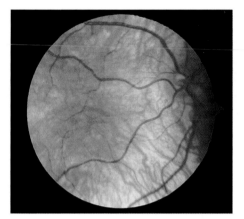

Figure 9-3 *Typical fundus hypopigmentation with readily visible choroidal vasculature in a child with albinism. Note pathognomonic foveal aplasia (lack of fovea and foveal avascular zone).*

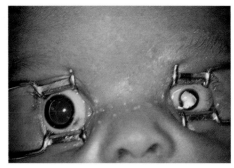

Figure 9-4 *This child has unilateral PHPV demonstrating leukokoria and severe microphthalmia (left eye).*

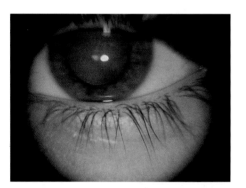

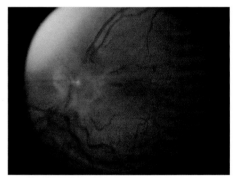

Figures 9-5 and 9-6 *Anterior PHPV with fibrous proliferation on the posterior lens surface (Fig. 9-5) and posterior PHPV with a regressed hyaloid vascular system and epiretinal membrane causing macular distortion (Fig. 9-6).*

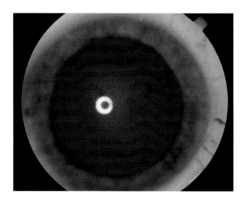

Figure 9-7 *Persistent hyaloid vessels surrounding the lens surface (findings diagnostic for PHPV).*

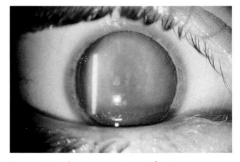

Figure 9-8 *An acute cataract due to spontaneous rupture of posterior capsule in a teenager with previously documented PHPV.*

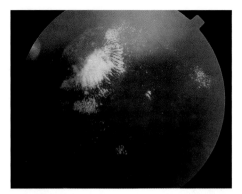

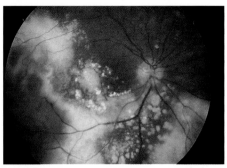

Figure 9-9 *This left eye of a young child with Coats' disease demonstrates dense lipid star in the macula and aneurismal telangiectasia of temporal retinal vasculature.*

Figure 9-10 *This photograph is from a patient with an unusual case of bilateral Coats' disease and optic disc neovascularization of the right eye.*

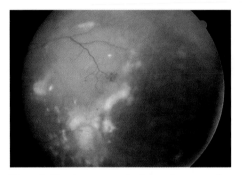

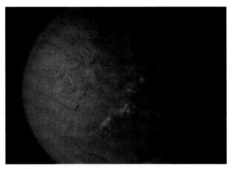

Figure 9-11 *A serous retinal detachment and vascular telangiectasia associated with a severe exudative response.*

Figure 9-12 *The typical "miliary aneurysms" of Coats' disease with surrounding serous fluid and lipid precipitates.*

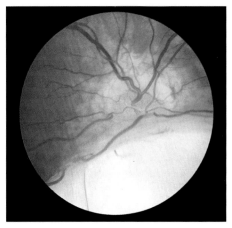

Figure 9-13 *A large, excavated chorioretinal coloboma inferior to the optic disc.*

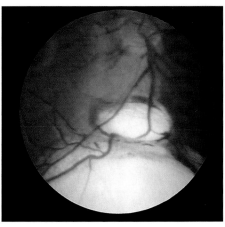

Figure 9-14 *Two colobomatous chorioretinal defects along the embryonic fissure.*

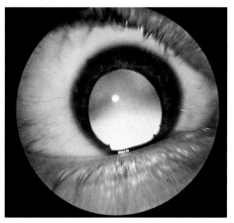

Figure 9-15 *Leukokoria caused by a large chorioretinal coloboma. Notice the inferior iris coloboma associated with this defect.*

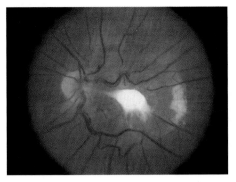 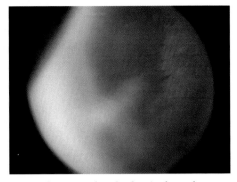

Figures 9-16 and 9-17 *A macular granuloma with associated epiretinal and subretinal membrane formation in a patient with ocular toxocariasis. This is a chronic lesion that has remained stable over several years of observation. Figure 9-17 shows the peripheral retina in the same eye as in Fig. 9-16 and shows granuloma with overlying fibrotic changes and adjacent pigment hyperplasia. (Figures courtesy of Alexander J. Brucker, M.D.)*

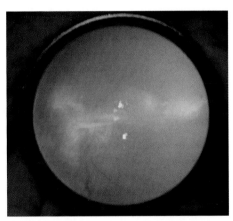

Figure 9-18 *The right eye of a child with FEVR showing posterior pole with lipid precipitates and epiretinal fibrous tissue.*

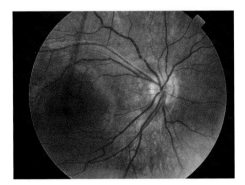 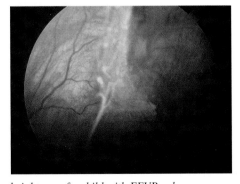

Figures 9-19 and 9-20 *Figure 9-19 shows the normal right eye of a child with FEVR, whereas Fig. 9-20 shows the peripheral retina of the left eye of the same child, demonstrating epiretinal membrane, lipid exudation, and peripheral nonperfused retina.*

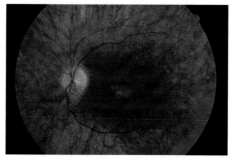

Figure 9-21 *The fundus photograph of a 22-year-old patient diagnosed with LCA at 1 month of age. Note attenuated retinal vessels and atrophic macular lesion. Peripheral bone spicules also appear at this age. At presentation in childhood, the patient manifested nystagmus, poor visual attention, and flat ERG. A lightly pigmented but otherwise normal-appearing fundus was noted. A mutation in the cone-rod homeobox gene was detected. (Photograph courtesy of Samuel G. Jacobson M.D., Ph.D.)*

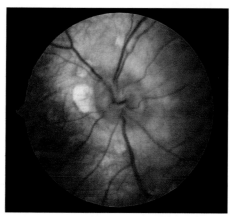

Figure 9-22 *The typical chorioretinal lacunae adjacent to the optic disc in an infant with Aicardi's syndrome.*

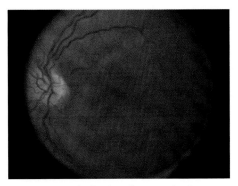

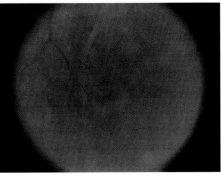

Figure 9-23 *The fundus photograph of an adult with X-linked retinoschisis and a bullous schisis cavity within the posterior pole. The patient has poor vision due to severe elevation of the retina involving the fovea.*

Figure 9-24 *X-linked retinoschisis with a peripheral schisis and subretinal bands along the margin of retinal elevation.*

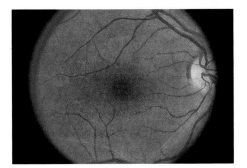

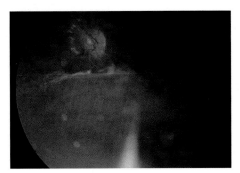

Figure 9-25 *The fundus photograph of subtle foveal schisis, a pathognomonic sign for X-linked juvenile retinoschisis. This condition appears clinically similar to cystoid macular edema.*

Figure 9-26 *A huge bullous schisis cavity involving the inferior retina of a child with X-linked retinoschisis who had multiple episodes of vitreous hemorrhage in this eye.*

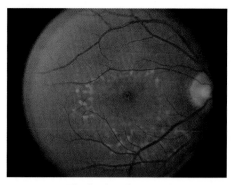

Figure 9-27 *The fundus photograph of a child with Stargardt's disease, demonstrating typical yellow pisciform lesions in the macular area. Notice that the foveal reflex is blunted.*

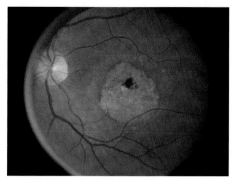

Figure 9-28 *The typical "beaten-bronze" appearance due to the atrophic macula in a patient with long-standing Stargardt's disease.*

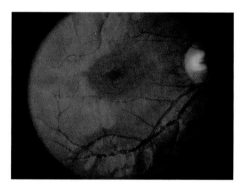

Figure 9-29 *The retina of an 8-year-old child with Stargardt's disease and poor visual acuity diagnosed 1 year before as "functional visual loss."*

SELECTED REFERENCES

Armstrong JD et al: Long-term follow-up of Stargardt's disease and fundus flavimaculatus. *Ophthalmology* 105(3):448–457, 1998.

Char DH: Coats' syndrome: long-term follow-up. *Br J Ophthalmol* 84(1):37–39, 2000.

Ebert EM, Mukai S: Familial exudative vitreoretinopathy. *Int Ophthalmol Clin* 33(2):237–247, 1993.

Erenberg G: Aicardi's syndrome: report of an autopsied case and review of the literature. *Cleve Clin Q* 50(3):341–345, 1983.

George ND, Yates JR, Moore AT: X linked retinoschisis. *Br J Ophthalmol* 79(7):697–702, 1995.

Lambert SR et al: Follow-up and diagnostic reappraisal of 75 patients with Leber's congenital amaurosis. *Am J Ophthalmol* 107(6):624–631, 1989.

Oetting WS: Albinism. *Curr Opin Pediatr* 11(6):565–571, 1999.

Pollard ZF: Persistent hyperplastic primary vitreous: diagnosis, treatment and results. *Trans Am Ophthalmol Soc* 95:487–549, 1997.

Tellier AL et al: CHARGE syndrome: report of 47 cases and review. *Am J Med Genet* 76(5):402–409, 1998.

Uchio E, Ohno S: Ocular manifestations of systemic infections. *Curr Opin Ophthalmol* 10(6):452–457, 1999.

OPTIC NERVE ANOMALIES

EDMOND J. FITZGIBBON

DEFINITION OF TERMS

The optic disc is approximately 50% of adult size at 20 weeks' gestation and increases to 75% at birth, reaching 95% of adult size at 1 year. The optic disc of the infant appears paler than in the adult, and the vascular pattern is somewhat more tortuous. It is useful to recognize and classify anomalous optic discs, since they can be associated with central nervous system (CNS) anomalies and genetic abnormalities. As a rule, bilateral optic disc anomalies present with decreased vision and nystagmus, and unilateral anomaly presents with "sensory" strabismus (usually esotropia). It is important to realize that amblyopia can contribute to poor vision in an eye with an optic disc anomaly, and a trial of occlusion is worthwhile.

DIFFERENTIAL DIAGNOSIS

MYELINATED NERVE FIBERS

This dramatic entity can present with a blurred disc margin that is sometimes confused with papilledema. Myelination begins at the lateral geniculate body at 5 months of gestation and proceeds distally, reaching the chiasm by 7 months and the optic nerve by 8 months, arriving at the lamina cribrosa at term. Intraocular myelination occurs in about 1% of eyes. Usually the myelination is continuous with the optic disc. It presents in the fundus as feathery white striated patches with irregular fan-shaped ends, partially obscuring the retinal vessels. It is bilateral in 17%–20% of affected infants. Visual acuity is not affected, although scotomas corre-

sponding to the area of myelination may be present. There is an association of intraocular myelination with myopia and amblyopia. Myelinated optic nerves can be familial, usually inherited in an autosomal dominant fashion (Figs. 10-1–10-3).

OPTIC NERVE HYPOPLASIA AND DYSPLASIA

This is the most common developmental optic nerve anomaly. The optic nerve is small, surrounded by a ring of hypopigmentation marking the end of an abnormal extension of retinal pigment epithelium and retina over the lamina cribrosa, and a second ring corresponding to the junction between the sclera and the lamina cribrosa (the double ring sign). Mild cases can be difficult to diagnose, and it can be useful to compare disc size to vessel size or to the disc to macula distance. Vision can be normal to very poor and is not well correlated with disc size. It occurs bilaterally in 60% of patients. Optic nerve hypoplasia is associated with CNS and endocrine abnormalities. Deficiency of growth hormone, hypothyroidism, diabetes insipidus, infantile hypoglycemia, and other endocrine abnormalities can occur. CNS malformations can occur, including absence of the septum pellucidum, corpus callosal hypoplasia, dysplasia of the third ventricle, and hypothalamic and pituitary abnormalities. The entity of septo-optic dysplasia or de Morsier's syndrome presents with poor vision and nystagmus due to optic disc hypoplasia, and short stature from growth hormone deficiency. Because of pituitary axis problems, these children may need supplemental corticosteroids in times of stress (Figs. 10-4, 10-5).

OPTIC NERVE APLASIA

This is very rare, nonhereditary, and presents as a blind eye without optic nerve or vessels. It is usually unilateral, and frequently other CNS abnormalities are present.

MORNING GLORY ANOMALY

This rare anomaly gives a large disc appearance. It consists of an enlarged, funnel-shaped, hollowed-out, and distorted optic disc, with a surrounding raised annulus of pigmentary disturbance and clumping. Often a central glial tuft is present. The vessels appear to radiate from the edge of the disc in a straight radial fashion and to be increased in number. Peripapillary arteriovenous communications are typically noted. Morning glory anomaly is most often unilateral. Although not hereditary, morning glory syndrome is associated with basal encephalocele, particularly if there is a V- or tongue-shaped area of depigmentation in the adjacent infrapapillary region. Serous retinal detachment can occur. Vision is usually very poor in these eyes.

OPTIC NERVE COLOBOMA

Colobomas of the optic nerve are caused by failure of closure of the embryonic fissure at 5 to 6 weeks' gestation. They can be unilateral or bilateral and are generally rare. Vision is often severely affected. The optic nerve appears large, with the retinal vessels distorted and widely separated as they exit the nerve. There is a sharply enclosed, white, bowl-shaped depression that occupies the large optic disc. This excavation occurs at the inferior aspect of the disc, and the inferior rim of the disc is attenuated. Colobomatous eyes may have myopic astigmatism. A serous retinal detachment can occur. Inheritance can be sporadic or dominant with incomplete penetrance. Optic disc colobomas are also seen in the CHARGE, Aicardi's, Goldenhar's, Meckel's, and linear sebaceous nevus syndromes (Fig. 10-6).

CONGENITAL TILTED DISC

This anomaly presents with an oval disc, typically with a depressed inferior side and elevation of the superior aspect. The optic nerve enters the eye at an oblique angle (Figs. 10-7 and 10-8). The scleral opening is larger than the size of the optic nerve head, creating a peripapillary scleral crescent. Vision is usually not affected, although visual fields can show bitemporal field loss that does not respect the vertical midline and is thus not associated with a chiasmal problem. Incidence is estimated at 3.4%, and 80% of tilted discs are bilateral. The retinal vessels emerge in a scattered pattern and not in normal arcades. Some tilted discs can have a "situs inversus" (Fig. 10-9) appearance because the vessels leave from the disc nasalward before turning back temporally.

PERIPAPILLARY STAPHYLOMA

This is extremely rare and usually unilateral. The disc, which is relatively well defined, is noted at the bottom of a depressed region. Vision is often decreased.

CONGENITAL PIGMENTED OPTIC DISC

A gray-appearing optic disc may be noted in premature infants who have delayed visual maturation and also can be seen in ocular albinism. True optic disc pigmentation is rare. The pigmentation is caused by melanin deposition in the anterior optic nerve or lamina cribrosa. Acquired optic disc pigmentation is seen in malignant melanoma and melanocytoma of the optic disc.

OPTIC DISC DRUSEN

Optic disc drusen (Fig. 10-10) are unusual in infants and most often present in the teenage years and tend to progress. The optic disc has blurred margins and is elevated, often with globular yellow-appearing excrescences on or below its surface. The overlying retinal blood vessels are not obscured, unlike in true papilledema. Optic discs with drusen tend to be smaller, not hyperemic, and the physiologic cup is absent. Often the optic nerve border is irregular and lumpy. The incidence of optic disc drusen is 0.34%, and in about two-thirds of patients they are bilateral.

Visual field defects occur, especially in the inferior-nasal region. Hemorrhages can occur, most often subretinal or below the pigment epithelium. Because the drusen are calcified, they appear on B-scan and CT scan. They also autofluoresce. Optic disc drusen are the most common cause of pseudopapilledema, particularly when the drusen are deep or indistinct.

OPTIC NERVE PITS (FIG. 10-11)

These are round or oval, typically olive-gray-appearing areas of the optic nerve head. They appear most frequently on the temporal or central aspect of the optic disc. Serous macular detachments occur in 60% of patients. Vision is usually normal unless there is a serous macular detachment, although arcuate scotomas may be present (Fig. 10-11).

PAPILLEDEMA

Disc edema can be unilateral or bilateral and have many causes, whereas papilledema is bilateral and due to increased intracranial pressure. In papilledema the disc is full and swollen with blurred feathery margins that obscure the peripapillary and surface retinal blood vessels. The optic cup is small and the veins are enlarged without spontaneous venous pulsations. Splinter nerve fiber layer hemorrhages may be present.

DOUBLING OF PAPILLA

Doubling of the optic disc is rare and most often unilateral. Typically there is a main disc and a "satellite," each with its own vasculature. The distal optic nerve is presumed broken into two fasciculi. An associated coloboma is common.

WORKUP

1. Complete developmental, pregnancy, labor, and delivery history
2. Complete ophthalmic examination
3. +/– Neurologic examination
4. +/– Neuroimaging
5. +/– Ophthalmic ultrasound
6. +/– Laboratory testing, e.g., blood sugar, pituitary functions
   Key: +/–, as indicated by history and examination.

TREATMENTS

1. Treat underlying neurologic and systemic conditions
2. Correct associated refractive errors
3. Treat associated amblyopia

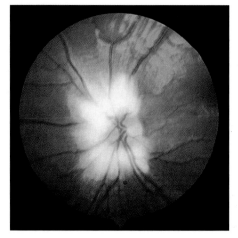

Figure 10-1

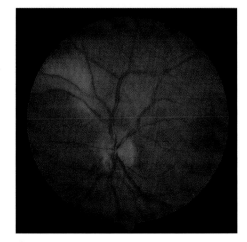

Figure 10-2

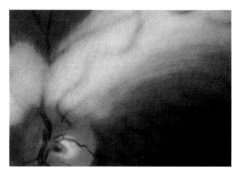

Figure 10-3

Figures 10-1 to 10-3 *The fluffy white striated pattern typical of nerve fiber layer myelinization. Note that the retinal vessels are obscured, and striations with a fanlike outer border are seen, especially in Fig. 10-3.*

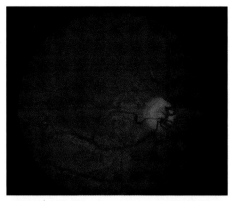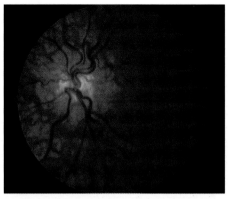

Figures 10-4 and 10-5 *Figure 10-4 shows a small central optic disc surrounded by a hypopigmented annulus that has a second hyperpigmented border (double ring sign) typical of optic nerve hypoplasia. Figure 10-5 demonstrates another small optic disc in a lightly pigmented eye with associated tortuous retinal vessels.*

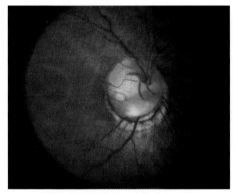

Figure 10-6 *A depressed glistening white region representing an isolated optic nerve coloboma in the inferior aspect of the optic disc with an associated thin inferior rim.*

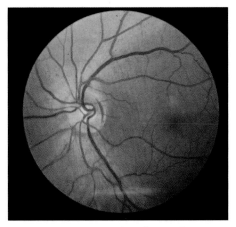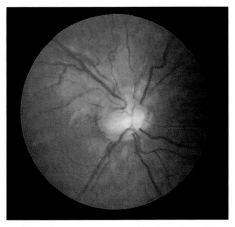

Figures 10-7 and 10-8 *These figures demonstrate optic discs that appear oval, with elevation of the superior margin and depression of the inferior disc. The vessels have an abnormal configuration and emanate nasalward, giving a "situs inversus" appearance to the disc.*

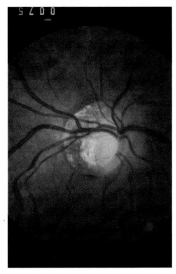

Figure 10-9 *An optic disc staphyloma, as shown by the relatively normal optic disc on the temporal aspect of a posterior excavated region.*

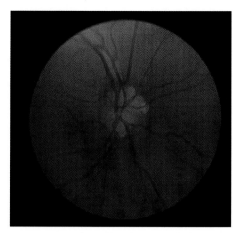

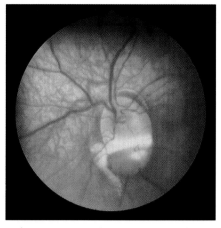

Figure 10-10 *Optic disc drusen with elevation, a "lumpy" appearance, and scalloped border from obvious drusen. Often in younger children the disc is elevated without evident drusen (buried drusen). One clue to help distinguish optic disc drusen from true papilledema is to appreciate the lack of disc hyperemia and obscuration of the optic disc surface vessels from nerve fiber layer edema that is always seen in papilledema.*

Figure 10-11 *An inferior optic nerve pit or isolated optic nerve coloboma.*

SELECTED REFERENCES

Brodsky MC: Congenital optic disk anomalies. *Surv Ophthalmol* 39:89–112, 1994.

Hoyt CS, Billson FA: Optic nerve hypoplasia: changing perspectives. *Aust N Z J Ophthalmol* 14:325–331, 1986.

Manor RS: Temporal field defects due to nasal tilting of discs. *Ophthalmologica* 168:269–281, 1974.

Pollock S: The morning glory disc anomaly: contractile movement, classification, and embryogenesis. *Doc Ophthalmol* 65:439–460, 1987.

Straatsma BR et al: Myelinated retinal nerve fibers. *Am J Ophthalmol* 91:25–38, 1981.

OPHTHALMIC INVOLVEMENT IN NONACCIDENTAL TRAUMA

CINDY W. CHRISTIAN and WENDY G. LANE

DEFINITION OF TERMS

Child abuse is a general term that describes acts of omission or commission by parents or other caregivers that are destructive to the normal physical or emotional development of a child. Child maltreatment includes physical, sexual, and emotional abuse, as well as child neglect. Child abuse results from a complex interaction of individual, family, and societal risk factors, and is legally defined by each state in the country. In all states, physicians and other healthcare professionals are mandated to report suspected abuse or neglect. Table 11-1 reports some statistics on child abuse and neglect.

DIFFERENTIAL DIAGNOSIS

1. Coagulopathy (ecchymosis)
2. Metastatic neuroblastoma with orbital involvement (ecchymosis)

Table 11-1 STATISTICS ON CHILD ABUSE AND NEGLECT

Reports to child welfare for investigation in the U.S.	3 million/year
Number of child maltreatment victims in the U.S. (reported and substantiated)	903,000/year
Number of known victims of physical abuse	200,000/year
Proportion of physical abuse cases with head and/or facial involvement	66–76%

3. Basilar skull fracture secondary to accidental injury (ecchymosis)
4. Forehead injury due to minor blunt accidental trauma (ecchymosis)
5. Other accidental injury (ecchymosis, laceration, burns, abrasion, fracture)

OPHTHALMIC INVOLVEMENT (FIGS. 11-11 TO 11-16)

1. Lid and external eye involvement, e.g., ecchymosis, laceration, abrasion, fracture of bony orbit, facial burns
2. Globe damage, e.g., conjunctival hemorrhage, chemical injury or instillation, hyphema, corneal clouding or scarring, glaucoma, pupillary sphincter tears, lens subluxation, cataracts
3. Vitreoretinal injury, e.g., retinal hemorrhage, retinal detachment, retinoschisis

DIFFERENTIAL DIAGNOSIS OF OPHTHALMIC INJURY

1. Accidental injury
2. Anterior segment dysgenesis
3. Herpetic keratitis (corneal scars)
4. Forceps use in delivery room (corneal clouding or scarring, hyphema)
5. Juvenile xanthogranulomatosis (spontaneous hyphema)

Cataracts

Metabolic disorders, congenital, inflammatory, syndromic, chromosomal, steroid induced (see Chap. 3)

Lens Subluxation

Marfan's syndrome, homocystinuria, syphilis, Weill-Marchesani syndrome, accidental injury

Retinal Hemorrhage, Exudates, Detachment

Hypertension, coagulopathy, infectious conjunctivitis, pertussis, severe cough, accidental injury

Vaginal birth (occurs in up to 40% of vaginal births)

Severe accidental trauma, intracranial hypertension with papilledema, vasculitis, meningitis, coagulopathy [e.g., leukemia, von Willebrand's disease, Idiopathic thrombocytic purpura (ITP)], endocarditis, sepsis, falciparum malaria, glutaric aciduria type I, following intraocular surgery, extracorporeal membrane oxygenation (ECMO) or general anesthesia, arterial aneurysm, arteriovenous malformation, Coats' exudative retinopathy, X-linked juvenile retinoschisis, *Toxocara* infestation, retinopathy of prematurity

EVALUATION AND WORKUP OF NONACCIDENTAL EYE INJURY

1. Thorough history and physical exam to identify circumstances of injury and to identify any additional injuries
2. Head CAT scan to identify presence of intracranial injuries, including acute subdural, subarachnoid, and intraparenchymal hemorrhage
3. Head MRI scan to identify presence of small extraaxial hemorrhage, parenchymal contusions, or old injury
4. Skeletal survey to identify occult fractures; this is mandatory in all children under 2 years of age; consider in children between the ages of 2 and 5
5. Complete blood count (CBC) and prothrombin and partial thromboplastin time (PT/PTT)
6. Abdominal trauma screen—Amylase and lipase measurements, hepatic function tests, urinalysis

MANAGEMENT OF NONACCIDENTAL EYE INJURY

1. Careful follow-up of retinal hemorrhages because of risk of visual loss in children with abusive head trauma; surgical intervention occasionally required
2. Mandated reporting to local child welfare agency if abuse is suspected

PROGNOSIS

1. Depends on type and degree of eye injury as well as associated neurologic injuries
2. Visual loss may result from cortical injury to occipital lobe, macular folds and scarring, epiretinal membrane formation, traction retinal detachment, and retinal tears

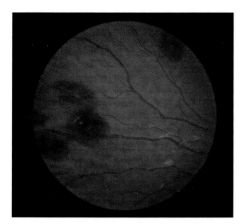

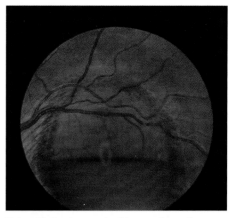

Figure 11-1 *Preretinal and intraretinal blot hemorrhages. Preretinal hemorrhages appear thumbprint-shaped initially, then may settle with gravity to produce boat-shaped hemorrhages. Blot hemorrhages are seen with deep intraretinal bleeding.*

Figure 11-2 *A preretinal hemorrhage that has settled to produce a large, boat-shaped hemorrhage.*

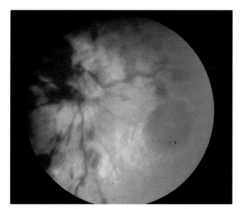

Figure 11-3 *Flame hemorrhages, which are seen with intraretinal bleeding into the superficial nerve fiber layer. Papilledema and a large preretinal hemorrhage are also present.*

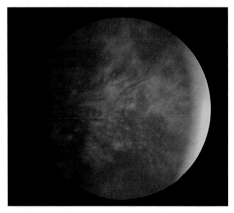
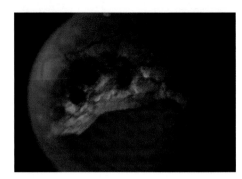

Figures 11-4 and 11-5 *Blot hemorrhages are again seen in Fig. 11-4; a fresh, very large preretinal hemorrhage is depicted in Fig. 11-5.*

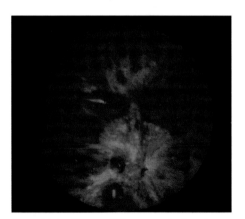

Figure 11-6 *Severe, diffuse preretinal and intraretinal blot hemorrhages characteristic of child abuse. Hemorrhages such as these are highly correlated with inflicted injury.*

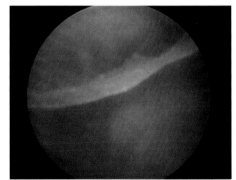

Figure 11-7 *A retinal detachment. Retinal detachment is an uncommon, but well described, finding in young children with inflicted head injury. Retinal detachments are associated with shaking injuries, but can also result from direct globe injury.*

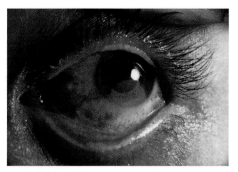

Figure 11-8

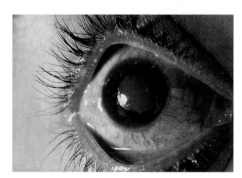

Figure 11-9

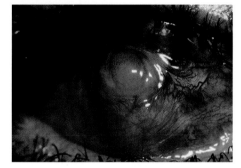

Figure 11-10

Figures 11-8 to 11-10 *Figures 11-8 and 11-9 are examples of conjunctival and corneal burns secondary to chemical instillation. The use of fluorescein confirms injury to the corneas in addition to the conjunctiva. Figure 11-10 depicts a subacute alkali burn to the conjunctiva and cornea.*

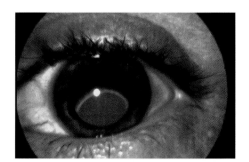

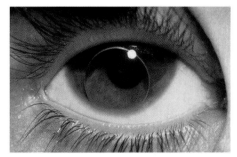

Figures 11-11 and 11-12 *These figures show dislocated lenses secondary to nonaccidental trauma. Lens subluxation in children is most commonly due to trauma. Unlike Marfan's syndrome, in which the lens is most commonly displaced upward, traumatic subluxation occurs in any direction but upward.*

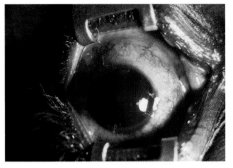

Figure 11-13 *The child depicted in this figure has a so-called 8-ball hyphema caused by direct trauma from a beating with a belt. The anterior chamber is completely filled with dark, clotted blood, causing elevation of intraocular pressure.*

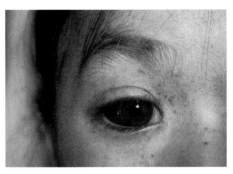

Figure 11-14 *A subconjunctival hemorrhage in a child who was assaulted by a neighbor, who also attempted to strangle the child. Periorbital petechiae are also noted.*

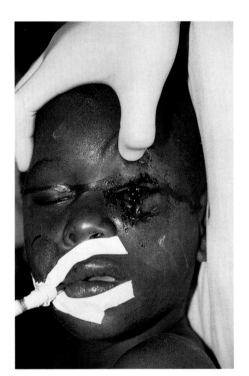
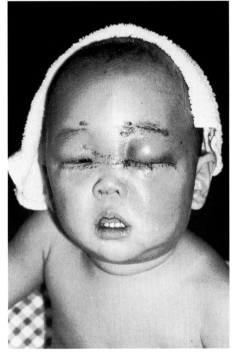

Figures 11-15 and 11-16 *These are examples of injury to the lid and external eye that may be caused by nonaccidental trauma. Figure 11-15 shows a lower eyelid laceration in a young child who was an unrestrained passenger in a motor vehicle crash. The driver had cocaine identified in a urine toxicology screen. Figure 11-16 depicts an infant with a left orbital cellulitis. The nidus of infection was felt to be abrasions around the eye, for which the parents had no explanation.*

OPHTHALMIC DISEASE IN INFANTS

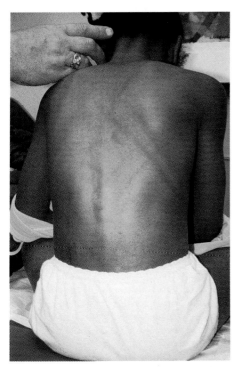

Figure 11-17 *A 5-year-old boy with multiple, long hyperpigmented loop marks from a beating with an extension cord. Patterned marks such as these are highly suspicious for abusive injury.*

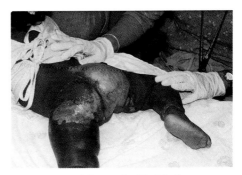

Figure 11-18 *A 9-month-old girl who was submerged in a sink of scalding water, resulting in severe partial-thickness burns. A skeletal survey revealed healing fractures.*

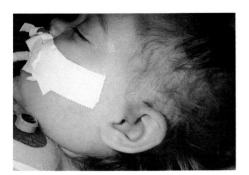

Figure 11-19 *A 1-year-old girl with the "tin ear syndrome," which describes unilateral ear bruising, ipsilateral cerebral edema, and retinal hemorrhages. Subdural hemorrhages are also found. The mechanism of injury is thought to be blunt injury to the ear that results in significant rotational acceleration of the head.*

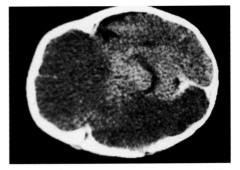

Figure 11-20 *The CT scan of a 15-month-old victim of abusive head injury shows an acute, posterior interhemispheric subdural hemorrhage typical of abusive head injury. In addition, there is loss of the gray-white differentiation of the right cerebral hemisphere and contralateral frontal lobe. Ophthalmologic examination revealed diffuse bilateral intraretinal and preretinal hemorrhages.*

SELECTED REFERENCES

Baum JD, Bulpitt CJ: Retinal and conjunctival haemorrhage in the newborn. *Arch Dis Child* 45:344–349, 1970.

Duhaime AC et al: Head injury in very young children: mechanisms, injury types, and ophthalmologic findings in 100 hospitalized patients younger than 2 years of age. *Pediatrics* 90(2):179–85, 1992.

Han DP, Wilkinson WS: Late ophthalmic manifestations of the shaken baby syndrome. *J Pediatr Ophthalmol Strabismus* 27(6):299–303, 1990.

Harley RD: Ocular manifestations of child abuse. *J Pediatr Ophthalmol* 17(1):5–13, 1980.

Jessee SA: Physical manifestations of child abuse to the head, face, and mouth: a hospital survey. *ASDC J Dent Child* 62(4):245–249, 1995.

Johnson DL, Braun D, Friendly DS: Accidental head trauma and retinal hemorrhage. *Neurosurgery,* 33(2):231–235, 1993.

Levin AV: Ocular manifestations of child abuse. *Ophthalmol Clin North Am* 3(2):249–264, 1990.

McClellan NJ, Prasad R, Punt J: Spontaneous subhyaloid and retinal haemorrhages in an infant. *Arch Dis Child* 61:1130–1132, 1986.

Naidoo S: A profile of the oro-facial injuries in child physical abuse at a children's hospital. *Child Abuse Neglect* 24(4):521–534, 2000.

Rubenstein RA, Yanoff M, Albert DM: Thrombocytopenia, anemia, and retinal hemorrhage. *Am J Ophthalmol* 65(3):435–438, 1968.

Sedlak AJ, Broadhurst DD: *The Third National Incidence Study of Child Abuse and Neglect.* Washington, DC, U.S. Department of Health and Human Services, Administration for Children, Youth, and Families, 1996.

Taylor D et al: The Ophthalmology Child Abuse Working Party, child abuse and the eye. *Eye* 13:3–10, 1999.

Weissgold DJ et al: Ruptured vascular malformation masquerading as battered/shaken baby syndrome: a nearly tragic mistake. *Surv Ophthalmol* 39(6):509–512, 1995.

Wilkinson WS et al: Retinal hemorrhage predicts neurologic injury in the shaken baby syndrome. *Arch Ophthalmol* 107:1472–1474, 1989.

NASOLACRIMAL DUCT OBSTRUCTION

SCOT LANCE

DEFINITION OF TERMS

Anatomic nasolacrimal duct obstruction is found in up to 30% of infants at birth, but only 6% of neonates are symptomatic enough that the family will seek medical advice for the problem. A relative narrowing of the distal nasolacrimal system resulting in decreased tear outflow is the most common cause of congenital dacryostenosis. Additionally, secondary nasolacrimal duct obstruction due to trauma, orbital tumors, and various developmental anomalies, including craniofacial clefts, may also be seen in the pediatric patient.

DIFFERENTIAL DIAGNOSIS

The most common manifestations of congenital nasolacrimal duct obstruction include

1. Congenital nasolacrimal duct obstruction (Figs. 12-1 to 12-6)
2. Chronic dacryocystitis (Fig. 12-7) (*Staphylococcus, Streptococcus,* and *Haemophilus influenzae* are the most common organisms.)
3. Acute dacryocystitis (Figs. 12-8 to 12-10) (*Staphylococcus, Streptococcus,* and *H. influenzae* are the most common organisms.)
4. Amniocele (Fig. 12-11)
5. Medial canthal encephalocele (Fig. 12-13)

WORKUP

1. Congenital nasolacrimal duct obstruction—Ocular and intranasal examination with dye disappearance test. These children have clear or mucoid discharge.
2. Chronic dacryocystitis—Gram stain plus culture and sensitivity of the punctal discharge if indicated by degree of purulence.
3. Acute dacryocystitis—Gram stain plus culture and sensitivity of the specimen obtained from the nasolacrimal sac at the time of surgery.
4. Amniocele (congenital lacrimal sac mucocele)—Ocular and nasal examination; ultrasound can be of value, as contact A scan and B scan show the amniocele to be a cystic space with low internal reflectivity.
5. Medial canthal dermoid—This entity usually presents not below, but above the medial canthal tendon. Workup should include observation and, if clinically appropriate, a CT scan.
6. Medial canthal capillary hemangioma—Ultrasound can be of value, as contact A scan and B scan show the capillary hemangioma to show greater reflectivity than a mucocele or amniocele. MRI or CT scanning will also help to differentiate these abnormalities.
7. Encephalocele—This mass will commonly present not below, but above the medial canthal tendon. The encephalocele will usually increase with Valsalva effects of crying or straining. A neurosurgical consultation is advised (Fig. 12-13).

TREATMENT

1. Congenital dacryostenosis—This can be managed conservatively because a majority will spontaneously open by 1 year of age. During this period, treatment includes properly performed lacrimal sac massage with the topical instillation of a broad spectrum ophthalmic drops or antibiotic ointment. In children over 1 year of age, probing and irrigation of the nasolacrimal system should be considered (Figs. 12-16 to 12-18). Silicone tubing is sometimes placed in a very obstructed system or in children who fail the probing.

Table 12-1 SELECTED MEDICINES FOR TREATMENT OF ACUTE DACRYOCYSTITIS*

Medicine	Route	Pediatric Dosage	Age and Dose
Erythromycin	po	0.5–1.0 g q6h	Children: 30–50 mg/kg/day (div q6h)
Cefaclor (Ceclor)	po	250–500 mg q6h	Neonates: Not recommended less than 1 month Infants and children: 20–40 mg/kg/day (div q6h)
Cephalexin (Keflex)	po	250–500 mg q6h	Infants and children: 40 mg/kg/day (div q6h)
Dicloxacillin (Dynapen)	po	250–500 mg q6h	Children: 25–75 mg/kg/day (div q6h)
Oxacillin	IV	1–2 g q4h	Neonates: 0–7 days: 50 mg/kg/day (div 12qh) 7+ days: 100 mg/kg/day (div q6h) Infants and children: 100–400 mg/kg/day (div q4h)
Cefuroxime (Zinacef)	IV	0.75–1.5 g q8h	Neonates: 10 mg/kg/day (div q12h) Infants & children: 50–100 mg/kg/day (div q8h)
Gentamicin	IV	3–5 mg/kg/day	Neonates: 0–7 days: 5 mg/kg/day (div q12h) 7+ days: 7.5 mg/kg/day (div q8h) Infants and children: 5–7 mg/kg/day (div q8h)
Chloramphenicol	IV	50–100 mg/kg/day (div q6h)	Neonates: 0–7 days: 10 mg/kg/day (div q12–24h) 1–3 wk: 20 mg/kg/day (div q8–12h) 3 wk: 30 mg/kg/day (div q6–12h) Infants and children: 50–100 mg/kg/day (div q6h)

*Consult manufacturer's product information for complete details before prescribing any of these medications.

2. Chronic dacryocystitis—The mainstay of treatment is proper lacrimal sac massage and broad spectrum topical antibiotic drops. If the infection persists despite massage and topical antibiotics beyond 2 weeks, probing probably will be required.

3. Acute dacryocystitis—If purulent material is obtainable with gentle compression of the lacrimal sac, obtain a Gram stain and culture with antibiotic-sensitivity testing. If not, surgical decompression of the lacrimal sac should be strongly considered. Initially empiric antibiotic coverage should be started pending the culture results. Pain control and the use of warm compresses are also to be considered. Neonates ad infants should be admitted for IV antibiotics. Table

12-1 lists selected medications for treatment of acute dacryocystitis.

4. Amniocele—The management is similar to that of primary nasolacrimal duct obstruction. However, because patients with this condition are at risk for acute dacryocystitis, probing is recommended if massage fails to collapse the amniocele.

5. Medial canthal dermoid—Surgical excision should be considered early if vision is an issue. If not, surgical excision can be delayed until a later age.

6. Medial canthal capillary hemangioma—Clinical observation can be the mainstay of treatment if vision is not an issue. Steroid injection and/or laser ablation can be considered.

7. Encephalocele—Combined orbital and neurosurgical evaluation.

CONCLUSIONS

Obstruction of the nasolacrimal drainage system may occur at any age but is a particularly common pediatric problem. Conservative management of primary nasolacrimal duct obstruction with diligent manual massage and broad spectrum antibiotic ophthalmic drops is usually successful. However, acute dacryocystitis in the neonatal or pediatric population is a medical emergency. This condition can quickly progress to orbital cellulitis or sepsis. Prompt diagnosis and effective treatment are essential.

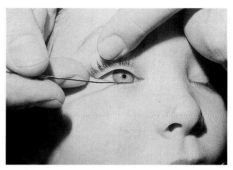

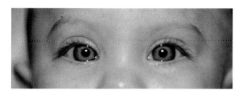

Figure 12-1 *A child with epiphora due to primary nasolacrimal duct obstruction.*

Figure 12-2 *The technique of probing the inferior canalicular system with a 00 Bowman's probe under general anesthesia.*

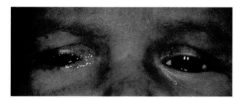

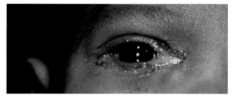

Figures 12-3 and 12-4 *Two infants with primary nasolacrimal duct obstruction and subacute dacryocystitis demonstrating a mucopurulent discharge of the right nasolacrimal system.*

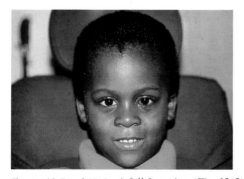

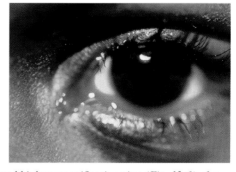

Figures 12-5 and 12-6 *A full face view (Fig. 12-5) and higher-magnification view (Fig. 12-6) of an older child with primary nasolacrimal duct obstruction and acute dacryocystitis with an enlarged, inflamed, left lacrimal sac.*

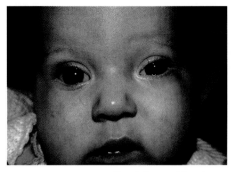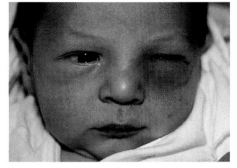

Figures 12-7 and 12-8 *Two infants with primary nasolacrimal duct obstruction of the left eye and an associated, mild (Fig. 12-7) and severe (Fig. 12-8) periocular cellulitis.*

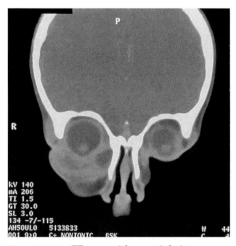

Figure 12-9 *CT scan with an axial view demonstrating a lacrimal sac abscess and associated periocular cellulitis of the right eye.*

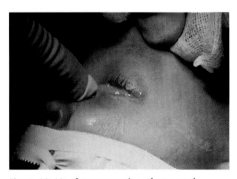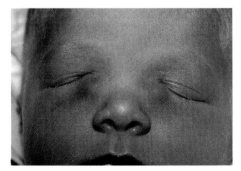

Figure 12-10 *Intraoperative photograph showing mechanical decompression of the left nasolacrimal system.*

Figure 12-11 *An infant with a bilateral amniocele of the nasolacrimal system. Note the characteristic bluish hue of the overlying skin.*

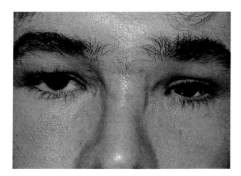

Figure 12-12 *A patient after extensive facial trauma with secondary nasolacrimal system obstruction on the left side.*

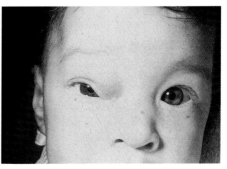

Figure 12-13 *An infant with an encephalocele of the right superior medial orbit causing ptosis and secondary nasolacrimal duct obstruction. Note that the mass is present above the medial canthal tendon.*

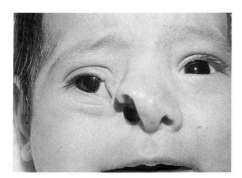

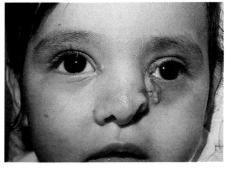

Figures 12-14 and 12-15 *These infants both have a form of facial clefting and secondary obstruction of the nasolacrimal system. Figure 12-14 is a right-sided cleft and Fig. 12-15 is a left-sided cleft with multiple skin tags.*

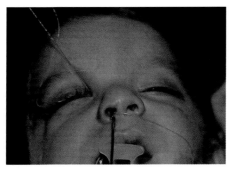

Figure 12-16 *Placement of Silastic tubes within the right nasolacrimal system under general anesthesia. This is used after unsuccessful probing and irrigation.*

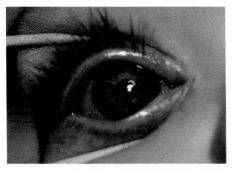

Figure 12-17 *An infant with the Silastic tube in proper position near the medial canthal area after it had been previously placed in the right nasolacrimal system.*

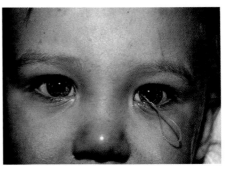

Figure 12-18 *A child with an extruding Silastic tube of the left nasolacrimal system.*

SELECTED REFERENCES

Baker JD: Treatment of congenital nasolacrimal system obstruction. *J Pediatr Ophthalmol Strabismus* 22:34, 1985.

Huber-Spitzy V, Steinkogler HJ, Haselberger C: The pathogen spectrum in neonatal dacryocystitis. *Klin Monatsbl Augenheilkd* 190:445–446, 1987.

Kushner BJ: Congenital nasolacrimal system obstruction. *Arch Ophthalmol* 100:597, 1982.

Linberg JV, McCormick SA: Primary acquired nasolacrimal duct obstruction. *Ophthalmology* 93:1055–1063, 1986.

McCord CD: The lacrimal drainage system. In Duane TD (ed): *Clinical Ophthalmology,* vol 4. Philadelphia, Harper & Row, 1986, pp 6–15.

Peterson RA, Robb RM: The natural course of congenital obstruction of the nasolacrimal duct. *J Pediatr Ophthalmol Strabismus* 15(4):246, 1978.

Powell JB: Nasolacrimal dysfunction. *Laryngoscope* 93:498, 1983.

Starr MB: Lacrimal drainage system infections. In Smith BC et al (eds): *Ophthalmic Plastic and Reconstructive Surgery,* vol 2. St. Louis, Mosby, 1987, pp 974–976.

Weinstein GS, Biglan AW, Patterson JH: Congenital lacrimal sac mucoceles. *Am J Ophthalmol* 94:106–110, 1982.

OPHTHALMIC DISEASE IN TODDLERS

AMBLYOPIA AND STRABISMUS IN TODDLERS

JOHN M. AVALLONE

Strabismus in toddlers and older children is similar in many ways to that in infants. The deviations in this age group may be more intermittent, and the association of monocular vision loss due to amblyopia is much higher. As in infants, strabismus is classified as either comitant or noncomitant. Children with noncomitant strabismus generally present with an occasional eye position abnormality, an abnormal head position (to gain the best eye alignment), or decreased vision due to the associated strabismic amblyopia. The most common diagnostic categories are briefly presented.

DEFINITION OF TERMS

AMBLYOPIA

Amblyopia is present in 2% of the population and is the leading cause of preventable visual loss in children. Strabismic amblyopia is the most common (occurring in 50% of patients with strabismus), followed by ametropic amblyopia (refractive, mostly anisometropia) and image-degradation amblyopia (lenticular and corneal disease are most common). The term *amblyopia* is from the Greek word *amblyos,* meaning "dullness of vision" (lazy eye). This is a neuropathologic process unique to infancy and childhood. It results in decreased vision in one or both eyes and is initiated by any condition resulting in abnormal or unequal visual input between birth and about 9 years of age. Normal and equal visual input is necessary (trophic) for proper cell growth and synaptogenesis of the postchiasmal visual pathways in the brain (lateral geniculate, visual cortex). Visual system cell growth and synaptogenesis are initiated at birth and are finished by 9 years of age.

If, during this period, one eye (or both) is not capable of normal and equal visual input, synaptogenesis and cell growth are disturbed, resulting in deficient vision. The younger the cortical vision system, the more sensitive it is to abnormal input. Amblyopia will develop after only 1 week of abnormal visual input in an infant less than 1 year old. The clinical rule is that a week of abnormal visual input per year of life is amblyogenic. The period of cortical visual development between birth and 17 weeks of life is the "sensitive," or critical, period. If a congenital or neonatal amblyogenic stimulus is not treated before the end of the sensitive period, it is impossible to recover full and normal vision.

Untreated amblyopia results in irreversible visual loss, with an increased risk of complete visual disability if the good eye is traumatized or affected by disease. Final visual acuity is dependent on the combination of amblyogenic factor, age at presentation, and compliance with amblyopia treatment. In general, the earlier the diagnosis and treatment, the better the prognosis.

Once the diagnosis of amblyopia is made, treatment is first directed toward reversing or decreasing the amblyogenic stimulus. Image-degradation amblyopia is treated by medically or surgically clearing the ocular media (lid hemangioma reduction, cataract extraction, ptosis surgery, corneal transplantation). Strabismic amblyopia is treated prior to surgery as part of the general treatment. This usually consists of a combination of spectacles and penalization. Ametropic amblyopia is first treated by giving the patient full correction of the optical error, either with spectacles or with contact lenses full time. As long as vision improves, no further treatment is needed (Figs. 13-1–13-4).

COMITANT STRABISMUS

Accommodative esotropia is convergent strabismus that most frequently presents at about 2 years of age. The synkinetic reflex of accommodation and convergence in the farsighted child most often causes this condition. (Focusing is coupled with convergence; in these patients, that connection yields the convergent misalignment.) The deviation is more apparent in the evening or with fatigue. The esotropia is often intermittent at first, or may be noticeable only with attention directed at a near target. In the office a near target with fine detail will help demonstrate the deviation. There may be a positive family history of accommodative esotropia. Treatment involves decreasing the patient's accommodation. Glasses are the mainstay of treatment; they may include a bifocal to decrease the crossing at near targets. Treatment may include miotic eye drops to change the relationship between accommodation and convergence.

The other common form of esotropia is "basic" esotropia without associated hyperopia. This often has associated "overaction" of the inferior oblique muscles, amblyopia, and a positive family history of strabismus. Glasses, penalization for amblyopia (patching or optical or pharmacologic blurring of the good eye), and surgery are the predominant forms of treatment, although some forms of "visual training" can be effective. Early treatment, especially during the intermittent phase, increases the likelihood of a good sensory outcome. Surgery is indicated if the deviation cannot be controlled with other treatment modalities. Comitant esotropia in this age range, as in infancy, may also be secondary to monocular vision loss, "sensory deprivation esotropia," or structural central nervous system lesions.

Intermittent exotropia is a divergent misalignment that may start in infancy but is most often recognized in older children. There is often a positive family history of strabismus. Unlike accommodative esotropia, where the intermittent phase is usually short-lived, the intermittent stage may last for years. The parent's chief complaint may be closure of one eye or squinting. This is seen most often when the child is outdoors or when he or she enters an area of bright light. The deviation may be seen only when the child is ill or tired. Of children with this disorder, 75% will show an increasing frequency and duration of the misalignment over time. As the deviation becomes more difficult for the child to control, it will become more apparent to professional and nonprofessional observers.

Treatment begins with correcting refractive errors and treating any amblyopia. Orthoptics ("visual training" designed to strengthen fusional control) to improve maintenance of fusion may be included in the treatment regimen. Orthoptics can be employed when the patient is of cooperative age and may be used in conjunction with surgery. Surgery to improve control of the deviation is the last step in the treatment protocol. The indication for surgery is poor control of the deviation.

Other forms of exotropia seen in this age group include sensory deprivation exotropia and exotropia associated with cerebral palsy or craniofacial disorders. In this age range, congenital esotropia patients who had surgery at an early age may present with "consecutive exotropia" secondary to poor binocular vision (fusional) control (Figs. 13-8–13-10).

NONCOMITANT STRABISMUS

As children mature, their demand for detailed vision increases and their head control improves. Strabismus that varies in different gaze positions (noncomitant) implies that one gaze position may have improved eye alignment over another. If a child has a gaze position that offers improved eye alignment, he or she will use that gaze position to achieve the best-quality vision. This may require an abnormal head position. Abnormal head positions in children are often attributable to strabismus. Discussion of some noncomitant strabismus conditions that may become apparent for the first time in toddlers and older children follows.

Superior Oblique Muscle Palsy or Underaction

The most common primary cause for vertical strabismus is a superior oblique palsy or underaction. This misalignment can be congenital or acquired. The palsy may be unilateral or bilateral. The acquired form is usually secondary to closed head trauma. The congenital form may present in the infant and child as an abnormal head position. The strabismus may not be due to cranial nerve disease, but rather to a long or lax superior oblique tendon. The patient will tilt his or her head and turn his or her face away from the side of the palsied muscle. The head tilt may be subtle or the child may manifest the posture only with visual interest. A persistent head tilt in infancy and childhood to adulthood will yield facial asymmetry and/or skeletal changes in the back and neck. Treatment may include prism glasses and patching for treatment of amblyopia. Surgery is often required for children with a persistent abnormal head posture (Figs. 13-11–13-14).

Duane's Syndrome

In 1905 Duane published a report of 54 cases of noncomitant esotropia with limited abduction of an eye associated with narrowing of the palpebral fissure of that eye on attempted adduction. The pathology is a congenital absence of the sixth cranial nerve on the affected side with aberrant innervation by the developing third cranial nerve. The narrowing of the palpebral fissure on attempted adduction of the eye is one of a number of key clinical observations that differentiates this condition from a sixth nerve palsy. The palpebral fissure changes are caused by co-contraction of the medial and lateral rectus muscles secondary to simultaneous innervation by the third cranial nerve. The ocular misalignment may yield an abnormal head position. This congenital condition has a predilection for the left side with a ratio of 3:1, left to right. It occurs in women 54% of the time. It is bilateral in 20% of patients. It is generally sporadic in its inheritance pattern. About 5% of patients will have a positive family history. Patients diagnosed with Duane's syndrome are 10 to 20 times more likely to have congenital birth defects than the general population. The defects associated with Duane's syndrome correspond to facial, ear, hearing, and upper thoracic and vertebral skeletal anomalies (Figs. 13-15–13-18).

Brown's Syndrome

Originally described in 1949 by Harold Whaley Brown, this syndrome is characterized by an incomitant vertical strabismus and an inability to elevate one eye in adduction. This condition may be unilateral or bilateral, congenital or acquired. The majority of cases are sporadic, although there have been enough familial cases to suggest some heritable predisposition. The eye will not elevate in adduction secondary to a tight superior oblique tendon or an abnormal tendon-trochlea complex. Acquired cases may result from trauma, infection, or rheumatologic disease. Brown's syndrome has been associated with rheumatoid and juvenile rheumatoid arthritis. The syndrome has also been reported with sinusitis and direct trauma to the area of the trochlea. Acquired cases may show tenderness and a nodule over the area of the trochlea. Children may present with an abnormal head position, with a face turn away from the affected eye, or a chin-up head position. In contrast to Duane's syndrome, Brown's syndrome is more often on the right side and affects males slightly more often than females. Treatment of congenital cases includes observation if there is a normal head position and no strabismus in functional gaze positions. Surgery is indicated if these criteria are not met. Treatment for the acquired cases may include observation or prescription of nonsteroidal antiinflammatory agents, and some authors support corticosteroid injections in the area of the trochlea. Evaluation and treatment of an underlying condition is necessary in acquired cases (Figs. 13-19 and 13-20).

Monocular Elevation Deficiency

Another more common cause for a noncomitant vertical misalignment of the eyes is monocular elevation deficiency. In contrast to Brown's syndrome, where the elevation deficiency is primarily in adduction, this condition limits elevation of an eye in all fields of gaze. Children with this condition may present with a chin-up head posture. The condition may be congenital or acquired. The congenital condition is far more common and may be caused by a tight inferior rectus muscle or a weak superior rectus muscle. Upper lid ptosis may accompany the elevation deficiency. There may be progression of the misalignment over time. Over half of these children will have amblyopia. Treatment includes addressing the amblyopia and the head position. A child with a significant chin-up head posture will require eye muscle surgery to improve the elevation of the affected eye (Figs. 13-21–13-23).

GENERAL WORKUP

1. History, with attention to family history of strabismus and refractive errors, developmental milestones, and general health and development
2. Ophthalmic examination; vision, eye alignment, sensory evaluation, external eye exam, dilated exam, and refraction

3. Laboratory, radiographic imaging, electrophysiologic testing or ocular motility recordings, and consultations based on ophthalmic evaluation

TREATMENT GENERALITIES

1. Correction of refractive errors, including the use of spectacles, bifocals, and miotic eye drops.

2. Orthoptics and prism glasses may be employed to improve control over eye alignment.
3. The treatment of amblyopia may include atropine eye drops, patching, and spectacles.
4. An abnormal head posture in children often requires surgery to improve the eye alignment and therefore the head position.

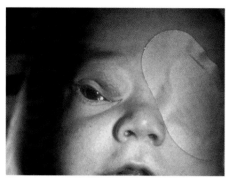

Figure 13-1 *An infant with visual deprivation amblyopia of the right eye due to an orbital hemangioma treated with occlusion therapy of the left eye (patching).*

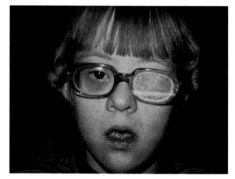

Figure 13-2 *A photograph of a child with refractive (anisometropic) amblyopia of the right eye treated with both spectacles and occlusion (patching) of the left eye.*

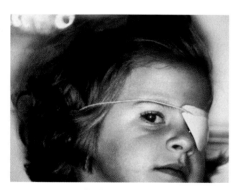

Figure 13-3 *A child who has been unsuccessfully treated for amblyopia of the right eye because she is able to "peek" with the left eye through this attempt at occlusion therapy.*

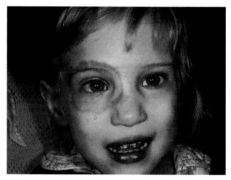

Figure 13-4 *A child with periocular skin inflammation or irritation of the right eye, a common complication of patching therapy for amblyopia. This is effectively treated with cessation of the patch and application of topical emollients and/or steroid-antibiotic ointment to the affected skin.*

OPHTHALMIC DISEASE IN TODDLERS

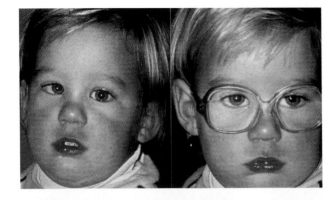

Figure 13-5

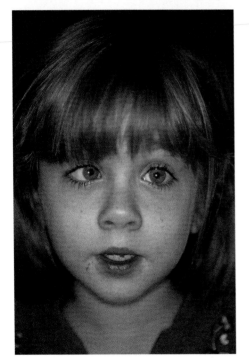

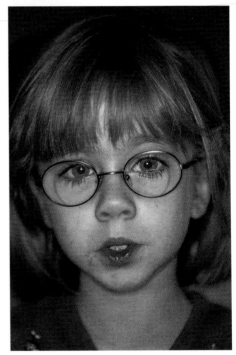

Figure 13-6

Figure 13-7

Figures 13-5 to 13-7 *Two children with accommodative esotropia, with and without spectacle correction in place. Without spectacles, the eyes are crossed; the left eye in both children is the preferred, fixing eye. With spectacles in place, the eyes are straight.*

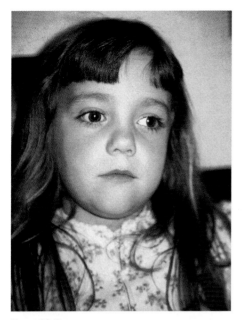

Figure 13-8

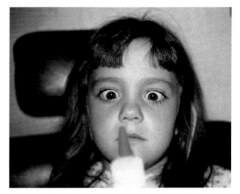

Figure 13-9

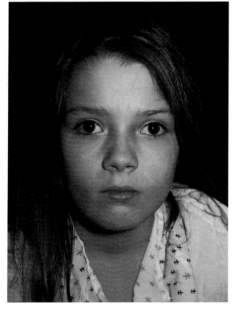

Figure 13-10

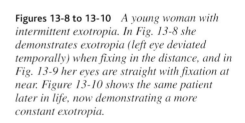

Figures 13-8 to 13-10 *A young woman with intermittent exotropia. In Fig. 13-8 she demonstrates exotropia (left eye deviated temporally) when fixing in the distance, and in Fig. 13-9 her eyes are straight with fixation at near. Figure 13-10 shows the same patient later in life, now demonstrating a more constant exotropia.*

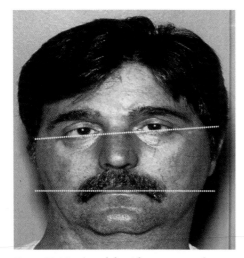

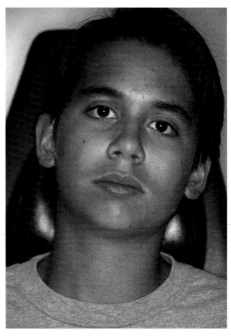

Figure 13-11 *An adult with an untreated, left congenital superior oblique palsy and the typical facial asymmetry associated with a longstanding head tilt. Two imaginary lines, one connecting the canthal areas of both eyes and the other connecting the corners of the mouth, are normally parallel to each other. As seen in this figure, the lines will intersect, indicating facial asymmetry.*

Figure 13-12 *A photograph of a young man with a typical head posture due to a right superior oblique palsy, paresis, or underaction.*

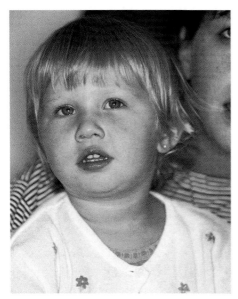

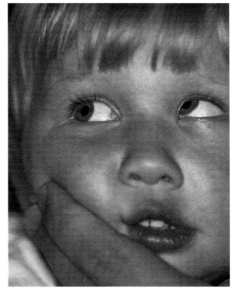

Figures 13-13 and 13-14 *The head posture and vertical misalignment in a child with a left superior oblique palsy. Note the left eye's "overelevation" in adduction due to the unopposed action of the inferior oblique muscle in Fig. 13-14.*

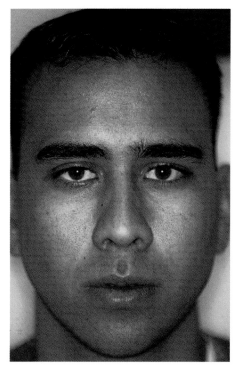

Figure 13-15

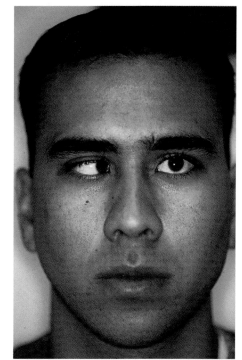

Figure 13-16

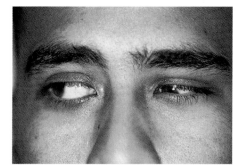

Figure 13-17

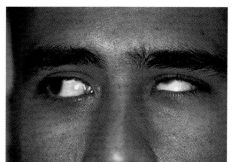

Figure 13-18

Figures 13-15 to 13-18 *A patient with Duane's syndrome on the left side with his eyes straight ahead (Fig. 13-15), during left gaze (Fig. 13-16), and during right gaze (Figs. 13-17 and 13-18). The patient's eyes are straight during gaze straight ahead (Fig. 13-15), but there is limited abduction of the left eye, causing esotropia in left gaze (Fig. 13-16). When the patient attempts to look to his right (Fig. 13-17), notice the narrowing of the palpebral fissure on the left side. Upshoots and downshoots of the affected eye are not uncommon in Duane's syndrome. This is illustrated in Fig. 13-18 by the overelevation of the left eye.*

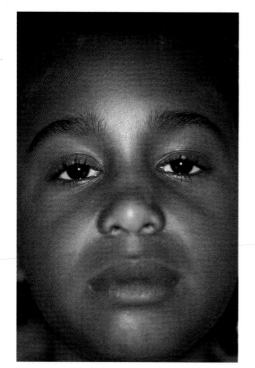 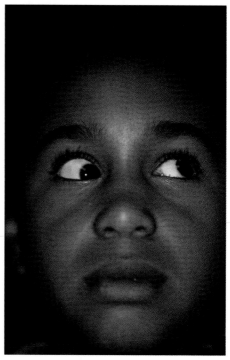

Figures 13-19 and 13-20   *These figures show a young woman with Brown's syndrome. Her eyes are straight when looking straight ahead (Fig. 13-19), but she has limitation of elevation of the right eye in adduction (Fig. 13-20). This causes a noncomitant* left *hypertropia.*

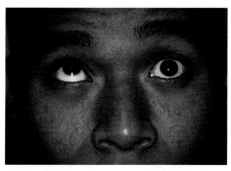

Figure 13-21

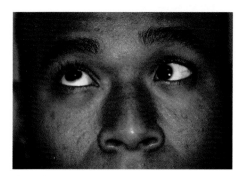

Figure 13-22

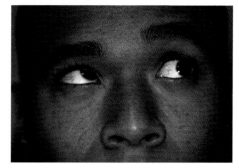

Figure 13-23

Figures 13-21 to 13-23 *This patient has a left congenital monocular elevation deficit. The patient cannot elevate the left eye in any position of gaze, e.g., straight ahead (Fig. 13-21), right gaze (Fig. 13-22), or left gaze (Fig. 13-23). This can be due to a hypoplasia of the superior rectus (and levator muscle complex) or to a congenital or acquired (trauma) "restricted" or "tight" inferior rectus muscle.*

SELECTED REFERENCES

Baker JD: Early onset accommodative esotropia. *Am J Ophthalmal* 90:11–18, 1980.

Ching FC, Parks NMN, Friendly DS: Practical management of amblyopia. *J Pediatr Ophthalmol Strabismus* 23:12–17, 1986.

Hotchkiss MG et al: Bilateral Duane's retraction syndrome, a clinical-pathologic case report. *Arch Ophthalmol* 98:870–874, 1980.

Hubel DH: Deprivation and development. In Hubel DH (ed): *Eye, Brain, and Vision.* New York, WH Freeman, 1989, pp 191–218.

Pfaffenbach DD et al: Congenital anomalies in Duane's retraction syndrome. *Arch Ophthalmol* 88:635–639, 1972.

Vaegan K, Taylor TD: Critical period for deprivation amblyopia in children. *Trans Am Ophthalmol Soc UK* 99:432–455, 1979.

Verecken EP, Brabant P: Prognosis for vision in amblyopia after loss of the good eye. *Arch Ophthalmol* 102:220–227, 1984.

von Norden GK: Mechanisms of amblyopia. *Adv Ophthalmol* 34:93–110, 1977.

Wilson ME, Eustis HS Jr, Parks MM: Brown syndrome. *Surv Ophthalmol* 34:153–172, 1989.

OPHTHALMIC INFECTIONS AND INFLAMMATION

EDWARD W. CHEESEMAN and DAVID B. SCHAFFER

DEFINITION OF TERMS

Conjunctivitis is an inflammatory condition involving the conjunctival surface of the eye. It is commonly divided into bacterial, viral, fungal, and allergic etiologies, although chemical insults (see Chap. 22) can also result in conjunctivitis. *Keratitis* is an inflammatory condition involving the cornea. It is characterized by edema, infiltrates, or necrosis of corneal tissue. In young children, trauma, preexisting corneal disease, and herpes simplex infection are the more common etiologies. *Blepharitis* is an inflammatory condition involving the eyelids. Common etiologies are the colonization of staphylococcal bacteria at the eyelid margin, seborrheic dermatitis, or lice that may attach to the eyelash margins.

Although it is easier to classify external ocular diseases by the specific anatomic structure affected, it must always be kept in mind that adjacent anatomic structures can commonly be involved simultaneously. For example, a *blepharoconjunctivitis* is an inflammatory condition that affects both the eyelids and the conjunctiva. Similarly, *keratoconjunctivitis* simultaneously impacts both the cornea and the conjunctiva.

Periocular cellulitis is usually classified as either *preseptal* or *orbital*. Preseptal cellulitis is characterized by an infection anterior to the orbital septum and needs to be differentiated from an acute *hordeolum* (stye), an acute *chalazion,* and true orbital cellulitis.

A hordeolum, or stye, is an acute, often painful localized bacterial infection arising either in a gland of the lid's tarsal plate or in one located around a lash follicle. With appropriate warm compresses as treatment, it usually comes to a point, ruptures, and then drains through the skin or conjunctiva or at the lid margin. A chalazion is a granulomatous reaction to the oil that has broken out of an inflamed meibomian gland. After a usually short acute phase, it becomes a slowly enlarging, generally painless mass in the lid. It usually has to be surgically incised.

Preseptal cellulitis is far more common than orbital cellulitis and is often associated with eyelid trauma or upper respiratory infections. Orbital cellulitis is a more serious condition that indicates that the infection is located posterior to the orbital septum. It is generally more painful and associated with severe lid swelling, proptosis, painful limitation of extraocular movements, and abnormal pupillary reactions.

Uveitis is an inflammatory condition involving the uveal tract of the eye (iris, choroid, and ciliary body). It may be anterior, posterior, intermediate, or a combination in its location in the eye. Uveitis is either infectious or noninfectious (see Chap. 18). Juvenile rheumatoid arthritis and juvenile spondyloarthropathies are common noninfectious (immune) etiologies for anterior uveitis in children. Sarcoidosis can commonly present as an anterior and/or posterior uveitis.

BACTERIAL BLEPHAROCONJUNCTIVITIS (FIGS. 14-1 AND 14-2)

DIFFERENTIAL DIAGNOSIS

The most common bacterial agents in children include the following:

1. *Haemophilus influenzae*
2. *Streptococcus pneumoniae*

3. *Moraxella catarrhalis*
4. Staphylococcal species

CLINICAL FEATURES

1. Mucopurulent discharge
2. Palpebral and/or bulbar conjunctival injection
3. Conjunctival chemosis
4. Often unilateral and no fever
5. Conjunctival papillae

WORKUP

1. History of associated systemic infection
2. Complete ophthalmic examination
3. Bacterial cultures and Gram stain

TREATMENT

1. Topical ciprofloxacin eye drops, 0.3%
2. Topical ofloxacin eye drops
3. Topical trimethoprim and polymyxin B eye drops
4. Topical erythromycin ointment
5. Topical tobramycin eye drops or ointment

CONCLUSIONS

Treatment of bacterial conjunctivitis and blepharoconjunctivitis is often empirical until culture results are available, except in cases where there is intercurrent illness or a hyperpurulent discharge suggestive of gonococcal conjunctivitis. With appropriate topical antibiotic treatment, resolution generally occurs within 5 to 6 days.

VIRAL BLEPHAROCONJUNCTIVITIS (FIG. 14-3–14-5)

DIFFERENTIAL DIAGNOSIS

The most common etiologies in young children are

1. Adenovirus (Fig. 14-4)
   a. Serotypes 3 and 7 cause pharyngoconjunctival fever (PCF)
   b. Serotypes 8, 11, and 19 cause epidemic keratoconjunctivitis (EKC) (Fig. 14-5)
2. Herpes simplex
3. Varicella zoster

CLINICAL FEATURES

1. Watery discharge
2. Often bilateral, although onset is not always simultaneous
3. Conjunctival hyperemia and chemosis
4. Preauricular adenopathy and fever
5. Follicles on palpebral conjunctiva
6. Associated lid swelling

WORKUP

1. Viral culture (if adenovirus or herpes is suspected)
2. Consider Giemsa stain of conjunctival scrapings (for *Chlamydia*)

TREATMENT

1. Supportive (cold compresses, topical decongestants).
2. Consider preservative-free, lubricating eye drops qid for comfort.
3. Topical antibiotic drops if secondary bacterial involvement occurs.
4. Some cases of adenovirus infections may require topical steroid or nonsteroidal anti-inflammatory drugs (NSAIDs).

CONCLUSIONS

Treatment of viral conjunctivitis is largely supportive, and the infection will usually resolve within 5 to 7 days. An exception to this is EKC (adenovirus), which can persist for as long as 3 weeks and may be complicated by subepithelial infiltration of the cornea or conjunctival membrane formation. Viral conjunctivitis is highly contagious, and the infected child should not be in close contact with others until the infection resolves. Strict hand washing should be performed by family members or other close contacts. This, unfortunately, can place some economic and logistical strains on busy families.

ALLERGIC CONJUNCTIVITIS (FIG. 14-6)

DIFFERENTIAL DIAGNOSIS

1. Insect bites
2. Toxic chemical reactions
3. Contact lens reaction

4. Graft-versus-host (Fig. 14-7) and immune reactions (Figs. 14-8, 14-9)

CLINICAL FEATURES

1. Acute, pale conjunctival edema with little discharge
2. No moderate or marked hyperemia
3. Usually bilateral (except insect bite reactions, which are often unilateral)
4. Watery discharge, light sensitivity, and marked itching
5. Follicles or giant papillae on palpebral conjunctiva

WORKUP

1. History of allergies
2. History of insect bites
3. Conjunctival scraping and staining for eosinophils

TREATMENT

1. Identify and remove offending agent if possible.
2. Systemic decongestants and/or antihistamines [diphenhydramine (Benadryl); loratadine (Claritin)] as needed
3. Local agents
   a. Decongestant and/or antihistamine drops (Prefrin; Vasocon A; Naphcon A)
   b. H_1 antagonists (Livostin 0.05% suspension)
   c. Mast cell inhibitors (Crolom 4.0% or Alomide 0.1% solutions)
   d. NSAID solutions [diclofenac sodium (Voltaren) 0.1%; ketorolac tromethamine (Acular) 0.5%]
   e. Corticosteroids (Decadron 0.05% ointment or Decadron 0.1% solution; Inflamase 0.125% or 1.0%; FML Forte 0.25% suspension)
4. Systemic desensitization to allergen if possible.

CONCLUSIONS

Treatment of allergic conjunctivitis varies considerably according to the severity of the child's symptoms and may require both systemic and local medications. Seasonal reactions will often have to be treated each year.

BACTERIAL KERATITIS (FIGS. 14-10–14-12)

DIFFERENTIAL DIAGNOSIS

The most common causes in children are

1. *Pseudomonas aeruginosa*
2. *Staphylococcus aureus*
3. *Strep. pneumoniae*
4. Fungi

PREDISPOSING FEATURES

1. History of antecedent trauma
2. Immune compromise
3. Contact lens wearer
4. Corneal dystrophies (development defects)
5. Prior corneal surgery
6. Recurrent herpetic infection

CLINICAL FEATURES

1. Pain
2. Photophobia and tearing
3. Conjunctival hyperemia and chemosis
4. Limbal flush
5. Cornea infiltrate and/or ulceration

WORKUP

1. History (including trauma and medication use)
2. Complete ocular examination
3. Corneal culture
4. Central scrapings for microscopic evaluation

TREATMENT

1. Topical ofloxacin 0.3% eye drops
2. Topical fortified antibiotics [tobramycin, amikacin, cefazolin sodium (Ancef), vancomycin)
3. Topical cycloplegic agents (e.g., atropine sulfate 0.5 or 1.0% solution)

CONCLUSIONS

Bacterial keratitis is relatively rare in young children and is invariably associated with some form of trauma or preexisting corneal or systemic disease. Prompt treatment is essential for the preservation of good vision in the affected eye(s).

HERPES SIMPLEX KERATITIS (FIGS. 14-13–14-17)

DIFFERENTIAL DIAGNOSIS

1. Bacterial keratitis
2. Herpes zoster keratitis
3. Recurrent corneal erosion
4. Resolving traumatic cornea abrasion

CLINICAL FEATURES

1. Pain, photophobia, tearing
2. Conjunctival hyperemia; limbal flush
3. Dendritic lesion of the corneal epithelium
4. Possible associated oral or blepharoconjunctivitis with cutaneous vesicles
5. Periauricular adenopathy
6. Ocular injection with watery discharge
7. Possible geographic lesion of the corneal epithelium
8. Decreased corneal sensation
9. If recurrent disease, corneal stromal involvement may be present

WORKUP

1. Fluoroscein or rose bengal staining of cornea to see dendrites
2. Herpetic culture of suspected lesions
3. Consider cultures for secondary bacterial invasion

TREATMENT

1. Topical antiviral medications [trifluridine (Viroptic) solution or vidarabine ointment five times a day]
2. Topical cycloplegics (atropine sulfate 0.5 or 1.0% solution)
3. Do not attempt to debride lesions in a child
4. Preservative-free topical lubricants
5. Consider oral acyclovir, 15 mg/kg per day, in divided doses for facial and other mucosal membrane disease and recurrent keratitis

CONCLUSIONS

Herpetic keratitis is often recurrent, with the virus inhabiting the trigeminal ganglion after the primary infection. The classic lesion is the epithelial dendrite, which is readily recognized with appropriate stains. Most patients heal within 2 to 3 weeks, but devastating corneal scarring may result from recurrent disease. Some children with recurrent disease may benefit from a maintenance dose of oral acyclovir for prophylaxis.

PRESEPTAL CELLULITIS (FIGS. 14-18 AND 14-19)

DIFFERENTIAL DIAGNOSIS

1. Chalazion or hordeolum (Figs. 14-20 and 14-21)
2. Dacryocystitis
3. Conjunctivitis
4. Allergic reaction
5. Orbital cellulitis

CLINICAL FEATURES

1. Generalized upper and lower lid edema with possible extension beyond the lids
2. Erythema
3. Pain
4. Possible conjunctival chemosis
5. Possible intercurrent sinus or upper respiratory infection

WORKUP

1. History of systemic illnesses
2. Complete ocular examination
3. Check specifically for normal ocular motility
4. Rule out evidence of proptosis
5. Consider CT scan to rule out orbital involvement
6. Gram stain and culture of any obvious wound discharge

TREATMENT

In a young child (<5 years), admission to the hospital for intravenous antibiotic therapy is indicated. Common organisms are *Staph. aureus, Strep. pyogenes, H. influenzae* type B, and *Strep. pneumoniae.*

CONCLUSIONS

Preseptal cellulitis in a young child warrants hospitalization for intravenous antibiotic treatment. Older children may be treated as outpatients with oral antibiotics and careful follow-up. It is important to make the distinction between this infection and the potentially more serious orbital cellulitis.

ORBITAL CELLULITIS (FIGS. 14-22 AND 14-23)

DIFFERENTIAL DIAGNOSIS

1. Preseptal cellulitis
2. Orbital pseudotumor
3. Thyroid-related ophthalmopathy
4. Cavernous sinus thrombosis
5. Rhabdomyosarcoma
6. Metastatic lesion to the orbit
7. Infiltrative lesion (leukemia)

CLINICAL FEATURES

1. Lid edema and erythema
2. Proptosis
3. Pain on eye movement
4. Possible double vision and/or abnormal ocular motility
5. Fever and possible headache
6. Possible afferent pupillary defect
7. Resistance to retropulsion of the globe

WORKUP

1. History of trauma, systemic illness, or immune defects
2. Complete eye examination to include pupillary response, motility, exophthalmometry
3. Check for decreased sensation in the V1, V2 distribution
4. Complete blood count and blood cultures
5. CT of the orbits, sinuses, and brain to rule out evidence of subperiosteal or intraorbital abscess

6. Culture and Gram stain of any discharge found from eye or sinuses

TREATMENT

1. Admit to hospital for intravenous antibiotics
2. Consultation to the pediatric and ear, nose, and throat (ENT) services
3. Tetanus booster for traumatic cases
4. Daily examination to monitor progress

CONCLUSIONS

Orbital cellulitis is a condition that warrants prompt hospitalization for intravenous antibiotics and very careful monitoring. Primary care for the patient should be by the pediatrician, with specialty consultation from ophthalmology, ENT, and possibly infectious disease. If an intraorbital cellulitis is noted on CT scan, then drainage is generally indicated.

INFECTIOUS UVEITIS

TOXOCARIASIS

Differential Diagnosis

1. Retinoblastoma
2. Coats' disease
3. Retinal astrocytoma
4. Recurrent toxoplasmosis

Clinical Features

1. White pupil
2. Possible associated visceral larva migrans
3. Usually unilateral
4. Associated chorioretinitis
5. Possible anterior chamber inflammation
6. Possible strabismus
7. Retinochoroidal granuloma

Workup

1. History (especially regarding travel and pets)
2. Complete ocular examination
3. Serum enzyme-linked immunosorbent assay (ELISA) for *Toxocara canis*
4. Consider anterior chamber aspirate for eosinophils (by ophthalmologist)
5. Ocular ultrasound or CT scan to rule out retinoblastoma

Treatment

1. Little known effective treatment
2. Consider steroids for the inflammation (p.o. or subcutaneous)
3. Antiparasitic agents have been suggested

Conclusions

Toxocariasis is acquired by humans through the ingestion of embryonated eggs of *T. canis* located in the soil. Unfortunately, there is little effective treatment for the disease. It is, however, extremely important to distinguish this condition from the life-threatening retinoblastoma.

RECURRENT TOXOPLASMOSIS

Differential Diagnosis

1. Syphilis
2. Toxocariasis
3. Tuberculosis

Clinical Features

1. Posterior uveitis with or without anterior uveitis
2. Yellow retinal lesion with vitreous cells; looks like "oncoming headlight in a fog"
3. Old chorioretinal scars with adjacent hyperpigmentation

Workup

1. History of raw meat ingestion or exposure to cats
2. Complete ocular examination
3. Toxoplasmosis-specific antibody titers
4. Consider human immunodeficiency virus (HIV) testing if history is suggestive
5. Test to rule out syphilis, tuberculosis, toxocariasis
6. Careful examination for secondary cataract formation

Treatment

1. Pyrimethamine and sulfadiazine with folinic acid supplementation
2. Clindamycin
3. Consider use of systemic steroids for associated inflammation

Conclusion

The exact nature of recurrences of toxoplasmosis is not clearly understood. Periods of parasitic reactivation may occur regularly and cause recurrent retinochoroiditis. To date, prevention of recurrent attacks has not been possible. If the macular region is affected, significant visual loss may result from chorioretinal scarring.

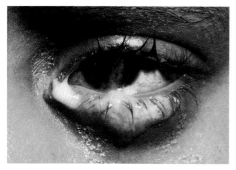

Figure 14-1 *The typical appearance of bacterial blepharoconjunctivitis with a dense mucopurulent discharge.*

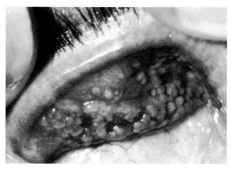

Figure 14-2 *This figure of the palpebral conjunctiva of an everted lid shows an intense papillary response typical of bacterial conjunctivitis.*

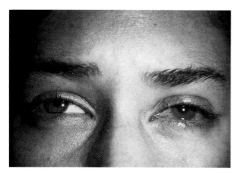

Figure 14-3 *Unilateral conjunctival hyperemia, chemosis, lid swelling, and watery discharge typical of viral conjunctivitis.*

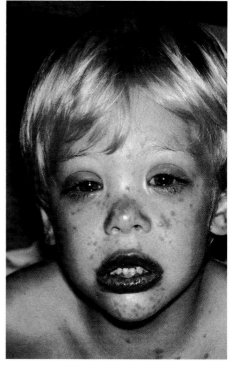

Figure 14-4 *The palpebral and bulbar conjunctiva of this eye involved in a severe form of adenoviral (hemorrhagic) conjunctivitis.*

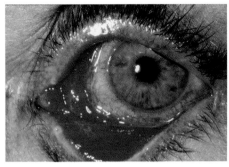

Figure 14-5 *The results of a highly contagious type of adenoviral conjunctivitis called* epidemic keratoconjunctivitis. *The immune-mediated keratitis associated with this viral infection of the conjunctiva is shown in the figure.*

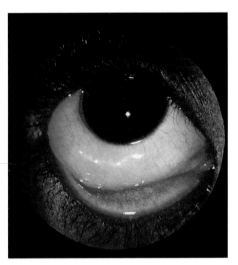

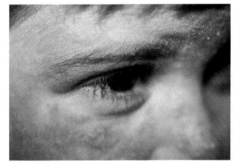

Figure 14-6 *The eye shows "bland" chemosis of the bulbar conjunctiva characteristic of allergic conjunctivitis.*

Figure 14-7 *This child has severe blepharo-conjunctivitis and dry eye due to graft-versus-host disease.*

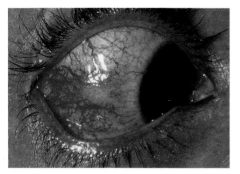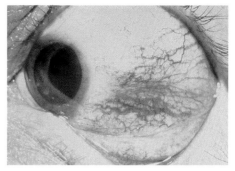

Figures 14-8 and 14-9 *The conjunctiva can be involved by autoimmune inflammations. Figure 14-8 shows isolated phlyctenulosis, occasionally a sign of tuberculosis, but now most commonly believed to be an immune reaction to staphylococci. Figure 14-9 shows a self-limited, idiopathic, localized, inflammatory process called episcleritis.*

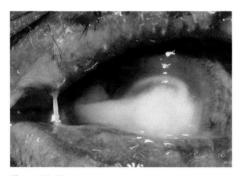

Figure 14-10

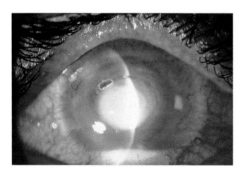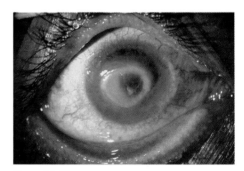

Figure 14-11

Figure 14-12

Figures 14-10 to 14-12 *Bacterial keratitis.*

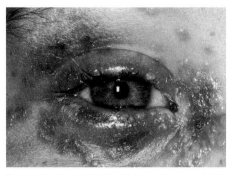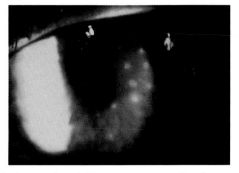

Figures 14-13 and 14-14 *Primary herpes simplex blepharoconjunctivitis appears as a periocular maculopapular eruption and can be associated with ocular mucosal and corneal involvement.*

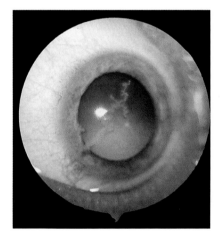

Figure 14-15

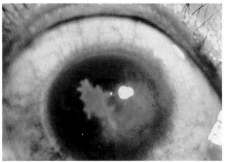

Figure 14-16

Figure 14-17

Figures 14-15 to 14-17 *Herpes simplex keratitis is a potentially blinding recurrent corneal infection. Fluorescein is retained by dead corneal epithelial cells in characteristic "dendritic" (Fig. 14-15) and "geographic" (Fig. 14-16) patterns. Repeated attacks of corneal infection can result in sight-threatening corneal scarring (Fig. 14-17).*

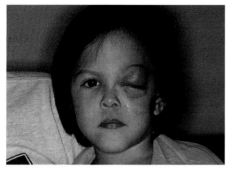
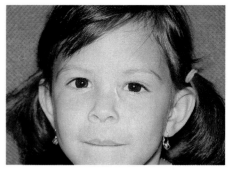

Figures 14-18 and 14-19 *Periorbital cellulitis can be a life-threatening infection and is often associated with paranasal sinus infection. Preseptal cellulitis is illustrated before (Fig. 14-18) and after (Fig. 14-19) antibiotic treatment.*

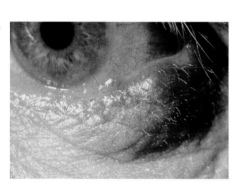
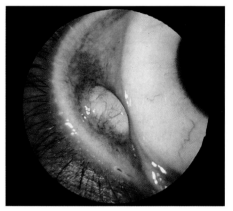

Figures 14-20 and 14-21 *Chalazia or hordeo-lums ("stys") are the result of obstructed meibomian glands (sebaceous glands of the lids). These are localized "sterile" abscesses and can spontaneously drain through the lid anteriorly (Fig. 14-20) or on the conjunctival surface posteriorly (Fig. 14-21).*

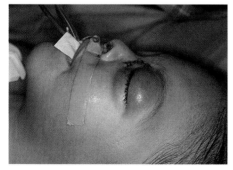
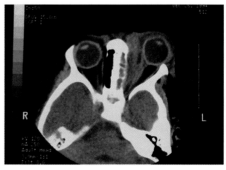

Figures 14-22 and 14-23 *Orbital cellulitis is shown in Fig. 14-22 with associated CT scan (Fig. 14-23) of the orbit, depicting inflammation in the medial orbit and neighboring ethmoid sinus.*

SELECTED REFERENCES

Ambati BK et al: Periorbital and orbital cellulitis before and after the advent of *Haemophilus influenzae* type B vaccination. *Ophthalmology* 107(8):1450–1453, 2000.

Block SL et al: Increasing bacterial resistance in pediatric acute conjunctivitis. *Antimicrob Agents Chemother* 44(6):1650–1654, 2000.

Bosch-Driessen, EH, Rothova A: Recurrent ocular disease in postnatally acquired toxoplasmosis. *Am J Ophthalmol* 128(4):421–425, 1999.

Clinch TE et al: Microbial keratitis in children. *Am J Ophthalmol* 117(1):65–71, 1994.

Cruz OA et al: Microbial keratitis in childhood. *Ophthalmology* 100(2):192–196, 1993.

Donahue SP, Schwartz G: Preseptal and orbital cellulitis in childhood. A changing microbial spectrum. *Ophthalmology* 105(10):1902–1905; discussion 1905–1906, 1998.

Ferguson MP, McNab A: Current treatment and outcome in orbital cellulitis. *Aust N Z J Ophthalmol* 27(6):375–379, 1999.

Gigliotti F: Management of the child with conjunctivitis. *Pediatr Infect Dis J* 13(12):1161–1162, 1994.

Mets MB et al: Eye manifestations of congenital toxoplasmosis. *Am J Ophthalmol* 123(1):1–16, 1997.

Nussemblatt RB, Whitcup S, Palestine A: *Uveitis, Fundamentals and Clinical Practice,* 2d ed. St Louis, Mosby, 1996.

Paivonsalo-Hietanen T, Tuominen J, Saari K: Uveitis in children: population-based study in Finland. *Acta Ophthalmol Scand* 78(1):84–88, 2000.

Pau H: *Differential Diagnosis of Eye Diseases,* FC Blodi and CF Blodi, translators. Stuttgart: Thieme Medical Publishers, 1988.

PTOSIS

DAVID E. HOLCK and JILL A. FOSTER

DEFINITION OF TERMS

Blepharoptosis is a unilateral or bilateral abnormally low position of the upper eyelid with the eye in primary position. It may be categorized by age of onset (congenital or acquired), or by etiology (pseudoptosis, neurogenic, myogenic, aponeurotic, mechanical). Congenital ptosis is usually noted at birth and remains stable. This condition is generally not inherited. Approximately two-thirds of congenital ptosis cases are unilateral. This condition may be associated with strabismus and anisometropia (refractive error difference between the two eyes). Up to one-third of the patients with eyelid ptosis will have corresponding superior rectus muscle weakness, and up to 12% may have anisometropia. If severe, this may induce amblyopia of the affected eye. Rarely, the ptosis will be severe enough to cause occlusional amblyopia.

In primary congenital ptosis the levator palpebrae superioris muscle is replaced by fibrofatty connective tissue. This results in a decrease in normal eyelid excursion and a lag in downgaze. Congenitally ptotic eyelids may present with a faint to absent eyelid crease. If the condition is bilateral, patients may have a compensatory brow or chin elevated head position (Figs. 15-1–15-11).

DIFFERENTIAL DIAGNOSIS

1. Syndromic association, e.g., blepharophimosis syndrome (6% of all cases of congenital ptosis). This autosomal dominant or sporadically inherited syndrome has associated eyelid findings of blepharoptosis, epicanthus inversus, and blepharophimosis.
2. Pseudoptosis may be caused by strabismus (especially hypotropia)
3. Orbital volume loss (after enucleation or orbital trauma)
4. Chronic ocular surface disease or intraocular inflammation
5. Neurogenic ptosis may be caused by cranial nerve III palsy
6. Horner's syndrome (ptosis, miosis, anhydrosis, with or without lighter-colored irides, especially in congenital Horner's)
7. Marcus Gunn jaw-winking phenomenon demonstrating a unilateral ptosis, which elevates intermittently with mastication
8. Myogenic ptosis is demonstrated by congenital ptosis (a localized developmental dystrophy)
9. Progressive external ophthalmoplegia
10. Myasthenia gravis, myotonic dystrophy, and oculopharyngeal dystrophy
11. Trauma
12. Toxic and acquired myopathies
13. Mechanical ptosis may be seen with eyelid and orbital tumors, eyelid edema, infection, hematoma, conjunctival scarring, eyelid skin diseases, brow ptosis, and dermatochalasis.

WORKUP

1. Complete eye examination (visual acuity testing is critical, pupillary evaluation, extraocular motility, anterior segment and fundus examination, and evaluation of eye protective mechanisms such as tear production and Bell's phenomenon).
2. Neuroimaging if central nervous system (CNS) or orbital pathology is suspected.
3. Occasionally, laboratory evaluation of pediatric uveitis (ANA RF), infectious process [computed tomography (CT), complete blood count (CBC), blood cultures], heritable myopathic process (muscle biopsy), myasthenia gravis [edrophonium

(Tensilon) testing, chest x-ray], or thyroid eye disease [thyroid function tests (TFTs)] may be indicated.

TREATMENT

1. The treatment of pediatric blepharoptosis is dictated by the etiology and degree of ptosis present, and the eyelid position's affect on visual function. The type of surgical intervention is chosen based on the degree of ptosis and, more importantly, on the levator function.
2. Any refractive error or amblyopia must be aggressively treated at a young age.
3. If vision is unaffected and the cosmetic deformity is minor, the patient may be observed until a later age.
4. Surgical treatment is warranted for visually significant ptosis. If amblyopia is present, surgical correction is indicated as soon as possible.

CONCLUSIONS

The treatment of pediatric ptosis begins with an evaluation of visual function, followed by treatment of any amblyopia with patching or glasses, and then surgical intervention to improve the function, level, or appearance of the eyelids.

Complications of no treatment may include amblyopia, permanent loss of vision, and psychosocial difficulties from the cosmetic deformity. Complications of surgery include under- or overcorrection of ptosis, eyelid contour deformities, poor eyelid crease formation, conjunctival prolapse, infection, scar formation, poor eyelid closure, lagophthalmos and exposure keratopathy, ectropion, and entropion.

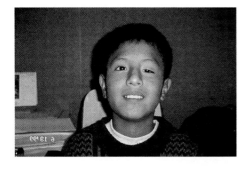

Figure 15-1 *A child with unilateral congenital upper lid ptosis having poor function of the left upper eyelid.*

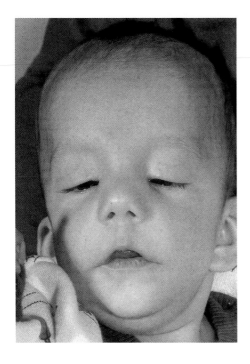

Figure 15-2 *A child with bilateral congenital ptosis and poor upper eyelid function.*

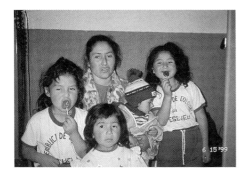

Figure 15-3 *This family with congenital ptosis has fair to poor upper eyelid function.*

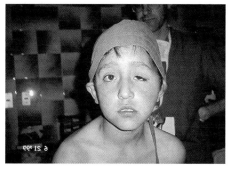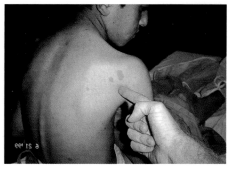

Figures 15-4 and 15-5 *A patient with neurofibromatosis and mechanical left upper eyelid ptosis secondary to a plexiform neurofibroma (Fig. 15-4) and associated café-au-lait spots (Fig. 15-5).*

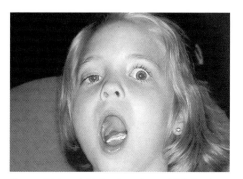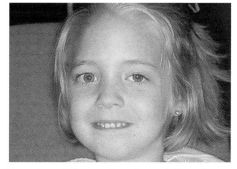

Figures 15-6 and 15-7 *A patient with left upper eyelid ptosis and Marcus Gunn jaw-winking phenomenon. Figure 15-6 shows the left upper eyelid retraction with use of muscles of mastication, and Fig. 15-7 shows the left upper eyelid ptosis with mouth closed.*

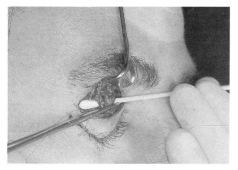

Figure 15-8 *The intraoperative view of fibro-fatty infiltration of the levator palpebrae superioris muscle in a patient with fair-function ptosis undergoing levator muscle resection.*

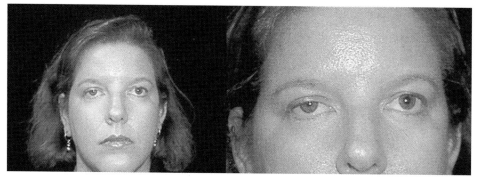

Figure 15-9   *A patient with congenital Horner's syndrome demonstrating ptosis miosis and lighter irides on the affected side.*

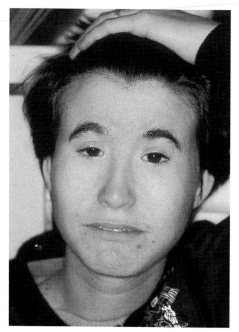

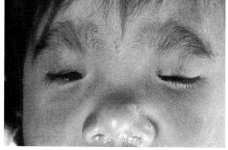

Figures 15-10 and 15-11   *This patient has bilateral ptosis associated with the blepharophimosis syndrome. Also present are blepharophimosis, epicanthus inversus, and epiblepharon.*

SELECTED REFERENCES

Clark BJ et al: Abnormal extracellular material in the levator palpebrae superioris complex in congenital ptosis. *Arch Ophthalmol* 113(11):1414–1419, 1995.

Engle EC et al: A gene for isolated congenital ptosis maps to a 3-cM region within 1p32-p34.1. *Am J Hum Genet* 60(5):1150–1157, 1997.

Fiergang DL, Wright KW, Foster JA: Unilateral or asymmetric congenital ptosis, head posturing, and amblyopia. *J Pediatr Ophthalmol Strabismus* 36(2):74–77, 1999.

Hornblass A, Kass LG, Ziffer AJ: Amblyopia in congenital ptosis. *Ophthalmic Surg* 26(4):334–337, 1995.

McCulloch DL, Wright KW: Unilateral congenital ptosis: compensatory head posturing and amblyopia. *Ophthalmic Plast Reconstr Surg* 9(3):196–200, 1993.

Mullaney P et al: The natural history and ophthalmic involvement in childhood myasthenia gravis at the hospital for sick children. *Ophthalmology* 107(3):504–510, 2000.

Willshaw HE: Congenital ptosis. *J Pediatr Ophthalmol Strabismus* 29(3):193, 1992.

ORBITAL TUMORS IN SCHOOLCHILDREN AND ADOLESCENTS

MATTHEW W. WILSON, BARRETT G. HAIK, and CHARLES B. PRATT

IDIOPATHIC ORBITAL INFLAMMATION AND ORBITAL PSEUDOTUMOR

DEFINITION OF TERMS

Idiopathic orbital inflammation and orbital pseudotumor are terms that refer to a heterogeneous group of nonspecific orbital diseases characterized by a polymorphous infiltrate composed of neutrophils, lymphocytes, plasma cells, macrophages, and eosinophils. In some patients, granulomas may be present. The diagnosis can be made only after known causes have been excluded. The onset of symptoms may be acute or subacute. Pain is a prominent feature and may be accompanied by lid edema, conjunctival injection, diplopia, proptosis, and decreased vision. Fever and malaise may be present. In children, a complete blood count may reveal a peripheral eosinophila (Figs. 16-1 to 16-4).

DIFFERENTIAL DIAGNOSIS

1. Orbital cellulitis
2. Thyroid eye disease
3. Ruptured dermoid cyst
4. Retinoblastoma
5. Metastatic neuroblastoma
6. Sarcoidosis

WORKUP

1. Complete ophthalmic examination
2. Magnetic resonance image (MRI) or computed tomography (CT) scan of orbit with intravenous contrast
3. Incisional biopsy

TREATMENT

1. Corticosteroids
2. Cyclosporine

CONCLUSION

Orbital pseudotumor is a nonspecific orbital inflammatory disease usually responsive to oral corticosteroids. An incisional biopsy should be performed to confirm the diagnosis and to exclude possible infectious causes.

CONGENITAL CYSTS AND DERMOIDS

DEFINITION OF TERMS

Dermoid cysts are the most commonly excised pediatric orbital tumor. Dermoid cysts are choristomas that arise from an epithelial rest of tissue trapped below the cutaneous surface, often near a bony suture. They are most often found in the superior temporal orbit along the zygomaticofrontal suture. Dermoid cysts may present as either superficial or deep orbital masses. Superficial lesions are usually noticed shortly after birth. They are usually asymptomatic, nontender, and well circumscribed. These do not normally threaten vision. Deeper lesions are located within the orbit. They may be adherent to the extraocular muscles or extend through the lateral orbital wall into the infratemporal fossa. Deep cysts may cause proptosis or a secondary strabismus. Undetected lesions may rupture after incidental trauma. Release of the enclosed keratinaceous debris may trigger a marked inflammatory response that may mimic an orbital cellulitis (Figs. 16-5 to 16-8)

DIFFERENTIAL DIAGNOSIS

1. Encephalocele
2. Mucocele
3. Microphthalmos with cyst
4. Teratoma

WORKUP

1. Complete ophthalmic examination
2. Ultrasound
3. MRI or CT with intravenous contrast

TREATMENT

Dermoid cysts should be completely excised. Epithelial remnants may form more cysts and further damage adjacent orbital structures. Care should be taken to avoid rupturing the cyst during excision, because release of the contents may incite a severe inflammatory reaction. If the cyst should rupture, the surgical field should be vigorously irrigated. The surgeon may also consider the use of depot or systemic cortico-steroids to quiet postoperative inflammation.

CONCLUSIONS

Dermoid cysts are the most commonly excised pediatric orbital tumor. Lesions should be removed intact.

VASCULAR TUMORS

HEMANGIOMA

Definition of Terms Orbital or lid hemangiomas may be purely capillary or mixed capillary and cavernous and result in lid deformity and proptosis. These tumors can interfere with vision by obstruction of the visual axis, causing visual deprivation amblyopia. They grow rapidly during infancy, with spontaneous involution in 70% of patients by 7 years of age. It is during infancy that these tumors pose the most risk to the eyes and orbits (Figs. 16-9 to 16-16).

Dilated and excessively numerous but well-formed capillaries in the dermis may be associated with Sturge-Weber syndrome. If the hemangioma involves the upper lid, there is a higher chance of associated globe involvement with glaucoma and choroidal hemangiomas (Figs. 16-12 to 16-16).

Differential Diagnosis

1. Lymphangioma
2. Varix
3. Dermoid cyst
4. Encephalocele
5. Mucocele
6. Orbital pseudotumor
7. Orbital cellulitis

Workup

1. Complete ophthalmic examination
2. CT or MRI with intravenous contrast
3. Ultrasound

Treatment

1. Corticosteroids—locally or systemically
2. Occasionally, surgical debulking or removal
3. Investigational use of interferon

Conclusions

Orbital and lid hemagiomas require accurate diagnosis of tumor extent and associated systemic findings. Continuous observation is needed to ensure normal visual development.

LYMPHANGIOMA

Definition of Terms Orbital lymphangiomas are proliferations of vascular tissue arising from an anlage of endothelial cells. Whether these tumors with endothelial-lined vascular spaces represent abnormalities of the venous or lymphatic drainage is debated. Scattered lymphocytes and/or well-formed germinal follicles may be found on histopathologic examination. The surrounding stroma contains hemosiderin and calcifications. These calcifications are visible on CT.

Orbital lymphangiomas most commonly appear during the first decade of life. Lymphangiomas are infiltrative lesions, which prohibits complete surgical excision. Periods of exuberant growth are intermixed with periods of relative stability. They show no tendency for spontaneous regression and are often associated with severe cosmetic and functional abnormalities. Lymphangiomas may be primarily conjunctival, subcutaneous, or orbital. Tumors of the upper eyelid produce a characteristic S-shaped contour. Involvement of the surrounding maxilla, mandible, and oronasopharynx may occur.

Dramatic changes in tumor size may occur rapidly, leading to marked proptosis. Reactive hyperplasia of the lymphoid tissue within the tumor may occur during an upper respiratory tract infection, causing marked enlargement. Bleeding within the tumor can lead to the formation of a so-called chocolate cyst and a rapid increase in size. An associated rapid increase in intraorbital pressure may compress the optic nerve, with subsequent visual loss (Figs. 16-17 and 16-18).

Differential Diagnosis

1. Varix
2. Capillary hemangioma
3. Plexiform neurofibroma

Workup

1. Complete ophthalmic examination
2. Evaluation of nasooropharynx
3. MRI or CT with intravenous contrast
4. Ultrasound

Treatment Medical therapy plays a minor role in the management of orbital lymphangiomas. Corticosteroids may provide a temporizing effect in tumors that enlarge following an antigenic stimulus such as an upper respiratory infection. Radiation therapy offers little help in the treatment of these lesions. Surgery remains the primary means of management for orbital lymphangiomas. Complete surgical excision is rarely possible due to the infiltrative nature of the lesions. Surgery is typically staged so that the results of each procedure can be assessed before additional excision is contemplated. The carbon dioxide laser ablates the tumor while providing maximal hemostatis. Cryotherapy can be used to disrupt cysts and sclerose vascular channels. Hemorrhagic cysts may be drained using a large-bore needle.

Conclusion Orbital lymphangiomas are infiltrating vascular tumors. Complete surgical resection is difficult. Management should be directed at minimizing functional abnormalities and cosmetic defects.

NEURAL TUMORS

NEUROFIBROMA

Definition of Terms Neurofibromas are benign peripheral nerve sheath tumors composed of a proliferation of Schwann cells, endoneural fibroblasts, and axons. Three types of neurofibromas have been described: localized, diffuse, and plexiform. Localized and diffuse neurofibromas are not normally associated with neurofibromatosis, whereas plexiform neurofibromas are almost always associated with neurofibromatosis. Localized tumors are well-circumscribed masses. Plexiform neurofibromas are diffuse infiltrating lesions that may have extensive involvement of the orbit, eyelid, conjunctiva, and periorbital tissues. Patients may present with a characteristic S-shaped abnormality of the upper eyelid, proptosis, decreased visual acuity, and strabismus.

Differential Diagnosis

1. Lymphangioma
2. Neurilemoma

Workup

1. Complete ophthalmic examination
2. Physical examination for stigmata of neurofibromatosis
3. MRI or CT with intravenous contrast
4. Ultrasound

Treatment Localized neurofibromas may be completely excised. Management of the diffuse infiltrative plexiform neurofibroma is more complex.

Conclusions Neurofibromas are peripheral nerve sheath tumors. Localized tumors are usually an isolated finding and may be completely excised. Plexiform neurofibromas are a hallmark of neurofibromatosis. Management is complex and requires multiple surgical procedures.

OPTIC NERVE GLIOMA

Definition of Terms Gliomas are low-grade juvenile pilocytic astrocytomas that may affect any part of the visual pathway. Tumors most commonly present during the first decade of life. Optic nerve gliomas are frequently associated with neurofibromatosis, type I. Lesions arising within the orbit are characterized by progressive proptosis, visual loss, optic atrophy, and unilateral optic disc edema. Tumors give a characteristic fusiform shape to the optic nerve on neuroimaging. Often there are kinks occurring in the anterior and middle portions of the tumor. The tumors can extend through the optic canal to the chiasm (Fig. 16-19).

Differential Diagnosis

1. Optic nerve meningioma
2. Sarcoidosis
3. Leukemia

Workup

1. Complete ophthalmic examination
2. Physical examination for stigmata of neurofibromatosis
3. MRI or CT with intravenous contrast

Treatment The management of optic nerve gliomas is both complex and controversial. These are benign lesions. Biopsy is discouraged because of the risk it poses to vision; thus, the diagnosis is based on the tumor's characteristic appearance on neuroimaging. Asymptomatic lesions may be followed with serial ophthalmic examinations. Enlarging lesions with decreasing visual acuity or that threaten the optic chiasm may be treated with radiotherapy. The role of chemotherapy continues to be debated. In patients with blind eyes, resection of the mass may be elected.

Conclusion Optic nerve gliomas are low-grade tumors diagnosed clinically. Management is controversial and should be tailored to preserve vision in both eyes.

PRIMITIVE NEUROECTODERMAL TUMOR (PNET)

Definition of Terms PNET is a neural tumor of childhood that is being recognized with increased frequency. It represents 4% to 17% of all childhood soft tumors. PNETs may either arise in the orbit or metastasize to the orbit. PNET is known to be a possible second primary tumor in patients with the hereditary form of retinoblastoma. PNETs are aggressive tumors that present with rapid proptosis and displacement of the globe. Destruction of adjacent bone may be seen on CT.

Differential Diagnosis

1. Rhabdomyosarcoma
2. Metastatic neuroblastoma
3. Metastatic Ewing's sarcoma
4. Osteosarcoma

Workup

1. Complete ophthalmic examination
2. CT or MRI with intravenous contrast
3. Metastatic survey

Treatment The management of PNETs includes an incisional biopsy followed by chemotherapy and radiation.

Conclusion PNETs are an aggressive neural tumor of childhood. Rapid progression is usually noted. Management includes biopsy, chemotherapy, and radiation.

FIBROOSSEOUS TUMORS

OSTEOMA

Definition of Terms Osteomas are benign tumors and represent 1% of all orbital tumors. They arise in the paranasal sinuses, the majority in the frontoethmoid complex. Osteomas are slow-growing masses that produce symptoms on the basis of sinus obstruction and intracranial or intraorbital extension. In some cases, orbital osteomas may be associated with Gardner's syndrome, a condition characterized by adenomatous polyposis of the bowel, colon cancer, and congenital hypertrophy of the retinal pigment epithelium. CT shows a round or lobular, well-circumscribed mass of bone density arising from otherwise normal bone.

Differential Diagnosis

1. Ossifying fibroma
2. Fibrous dysplasia
3. Giant cell tumor
4. Osteosarcoma
5. Chondroma
6. Chondrosarcoma

Workup

1. Complete ophthalmic examination
2. Systemic examination for Gardner's syndrome
3. CT with intravenous contrast

Treatment Small osteomas may be observed. Larger lesions that threaten vision should be completely excised.

Conclusion Osteomas are slow-growing benign tumors. Small lesions may be observed, whereas larger tumors are best excised. Patients should be evaluated for Gardner's syndrome.

FIBROUS DYSPLASIA

Definition of Terms Fibrous dysplasia is a fibroosseous lesion occurring most often in the first and second decades of life. It results from an idiopathic arrest in the normal maturation of bone, leaving a highly vascularized woven bone rather than the normal compact bone. Fibrous dysplasia most often affects the frontal bone, resulting in proptosis and downward displacement of the globe. Expanding lesions encroach on the optic canal, leading to a decrease in visual acuity. Fibrous dysplasia may be monostotic or polyostotic, with the latter being associated with Albright's syndrome. Most orbital lesions are monostotic. Fibrous dysplasia may undergo malignant transformation into either osteosarcoma or fibrosarcoma.

Differential Diagnosis

1. Ossifying fibroma
2. Osteoma
3. Giant cell tumor
4. Osteosarcoma
5. Chondroma
6. Chondrosarcoma

Workup

1. Complete ophthalmic examination
2. CT with intravenous contrast

Treatment Observation is recommended for non-vision-threatening lesions. Fibrous dysplasia may remain stable for years. In cases where vision is threatened, decompression of the optic canal via a neurosurgical approach may be needed. Cosmetically unacceptable lesions may also be resected in combination with craniofacial reconstruction.

Conclusions Fibrous dysplasia results from an abnormality of bone development. Monostotic lesions most frequently affect the orbit. Patients should be monitored closely for evidence of optic nerve compression. Surgical resection requires a multidisciplinary team composed of an orbital surgeon, neurosurgeon, and otolaryngologist.

OSTEOSARCOMA

Definition of Terms Osteosarcoma is the most common primary malignant neoplasm of bone. The majority of tumors arise de novo, but some occur secondary to irradiation or predisposing conditions such as the hereditary form of retinoblastoma. Osteosarcomas usually occur during the second decade of life. Orbital involvement results most often from maxillary disease. Symptoms include proptosis, vertical displacement of the globe, pain, periorbital numbness, eyelid edema, and conjunctival chemosis. CT shows bony lytic and sclerotic changes with adjacent soft tissue infiltration. Focal areas of calcification may be seen. Serum alkaline phosphatase levels may be elevated.

Differential Diagnosis

1. Fibrous dysplasia
2. Paget's disease
3. Ossifying fibroma
4. Osteoma
5. Giant cell tumor
6. Chondroma
7. Chondrosarcoma

Workup

1. Complete ophthalmic examination
2. CT with intravenous contrast

Treatment The management of osteosarcoma is complete surgical resection combined with radiation and chemotherapy.

Conclusion Osteosarcoma is a high-grade bony malignancy that most often arises de novo, but is more commonly thought of as a second malignancy in patients with the hereditary form of retinoblastoma. Management involves surgery, chemotherapy, and radiation.

MYOGENIC TUMORS

RHABDOMYOSARCOMA

Definition of Terms Rhabdomyosarcoma is the most common primary orbital malignancy of childhood, accounting for approximately 1%

of all orbital tumors. Rhabdomyosarcoma presents during the first two decades of life as a rapidly enlarging orbital mass. Tumors may arise in either the orbit or the paranasal sinuses. Orbital rhabdomyosarcoma has been reported as a secondary malignancy following irradiation for the treatment of retinoblastoma. Symptoms include proptosis, vertical displacement of the globe, and conjunctival chemosis. Clinicians should entertain this diagnosis in the setting of suspected orbital trauma and non-resolving orbital cellulitis (Fig. 16-20).

Differential Diagnosis

1. Orbital cellulitis
2. Orbital trauma
3. Leiomyosarcoma
4. Idiopathic orbital inflammation

Workup

1. Complete ophthalmic examination
2. MRI or CT with intravenous contrast
3. Bone marrow biopsy or aspirate
4. Lumbar puncture
5. Bone scan

Treatment Surgery should be limited to an incisional biopsy without mutilation of orbital structures followed by radiotherapy and chemotherapy. Survival rates have dramatically improved using this treatment strategy.

Conclusion Rhabdomyosarcoma is the most common orbital malignancy of childhood. Surgery should be limited to a confirmatory biopsy. Radiotherapy and chemotherapy are highly effective in treating this disease.

LYMPHOID, LEUKEMIC, AND HISTIOCYTIC TUMORS

LEUKEMIA

Definition of Terms All forms of leukemia may affect the orbit. Orbital involvement is more common with the acute rather the chronic forms of the disease. The most common orbital presentation in children is the chloroma or granulocytic sarcoma, which results from the invasion of the soft tissues by an acute myelogenous leukemia. Chloromas are a frequent cause of unilateral proptosis in children. Onset is often rapid and may be the initial manifestation of the disease. Bilateral involvement may occur. Children with leukemia are subject to spontaneous

orbital hemorrhages with rapid proptosis and visual compromise (Fig. 16-21).

Differential Diagnosis

1. Orbital cellulitis
2. Hemorrhage
3. Rhabdomyosarcoma
4. Metastatic neuroblastoma

Workup

1. Complete ophthalmic examination
2. MRI or CT with intravenous contrast
3. Ultrasound

Treatment In patients who have no history of malignancy, a biopsy should be performed to establish the diagnosis. Management should address the systemic nature of the disease. The leukemic infiltrate is sensitive to chemotherapy. If the optic nerve or vision is threatened, local radiation may be used to achieve a faster response.

Conclusions Leukemia may invade the orbit. The chloroma or granulocytic sarcoma is the most common pediatric orbital manifestation. Lesions are sensitive to chemotherapy. In cases where vision is threatened, radiation should be considered.

LANGERHANS' CELL HISTIOCYTOSIS

Definition of Terms Langerhans' cell histiocytosis is now the accepted name for a spectrum of diseases which include histiocytosis X, eosinophilic granuloma, Hand-Schüller-Christian disease, and Letterer-Siwe disease. Orbital involvement usually occurs as a solitary bone lesion and has been previously referred to as eosinophilic granuloma. Patients typically present within the first decade of life with edema of the upper eyelid. The lesions are most often located superotemporally. Pain, redness, and tenderness are common findings. CT shows a lytic bone lesion involving the frontal or zygomatic bone. MRI provides greater detail of the soft tissue involvement.

Differential Diagnosis

1. Orbital cellulitis
2. Orbital pseudotumor
3. Dacryoadenitis
4. Ruptured dermoid cyst
5. Metastatic neuroblastoma

Workup

1. Complete ophthalmic examination
2. CT or MRI
3. Systemic evaluation to exclude other foci of disease

Treatment Management of the lesions includes biopsy followed by curettage of the bone. Systemic or local steroids may be used. In some cases, chemotherapy and/or low-dose radiation may be needed.

Conclusions Langerhans' cell histiocytosis may present as localized or diffuse disease. Orbital involvement is typically limited to a solitary orbital bony lesion without systemic involvement. Most orbital lesions can be treated by local measures.

SECONDARY OR METASTATIC TUMORS

NEUROBLASTOMA

Definition of Terms Neuroblastoma is the second most common malignant orbital tumor of childhood. Orbital neuroblastoma most often represents a metastasis from an abdominal, thoracic, or pelvic primary. However, in rare cases neuroblastoma may arise in the orbit. The orbital presentation of metastatic neuroblastoma is characterized by the sudden onset of proptosis, periorbital swelling, ptosis, and ecchymosis. Other ophthalmic findings may include a Horner's syndrome and opsoclonus. Approximately 40% of the patients will have bilateral orbital disease. CT may show evidence of bony destruction and other cranial metastases.

Differential Diagnosis

1. Orbital cellulitis
2. Orbital pseudotumor
3. Rhabdomyosarcoma
4. Metastatic Ewing's sarcoma
5. Primitive neuroectodermal tumor

Workup

1. Complete ophthalmic examination
2. CT or MRI with intravenous contrast

Treatment A biopsy may be performed to confirm the diagnosis. Chemotherapy is still an effective means of treating systemic disease. Radiation may be needed if vision or the optic nerve is threatened. Investigational studies are underway to explore the use of vaccines in the treatment of metastatic disease.

Conclusion Metastatic neuroblastoma is the second most common malignant tumor of the pediatric orbit. Disease progression is rapid and often mimics an inflammatory disease. Chemotherapy and possible radiation are the mainstays of treatment.

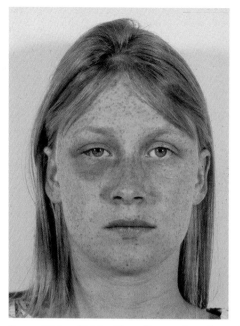

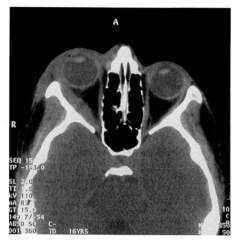

Figures 16-1 and 16-2   *These figures show the periocular inflammation (Fig. 16-1) and typical CT scan (Fig. 16-2) appearance of idiopathic orbital inflammation. The CT scan shows diffuse swelling of the right lateral rectus, including the tendon.*

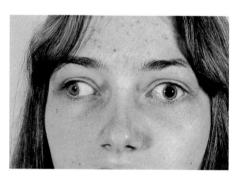

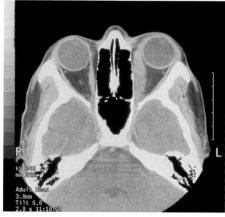

Figures 16-3 and 16-4   *This young woman has proptosis and paralytic strabismus (exotropia) with inflammation of the conjunctiva (Fig. 16-3) due to inflammatory myositis of her left medial rectus as seen by the CT scan in Fig. 16-4.*

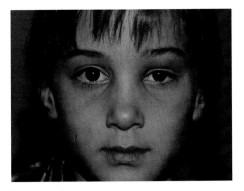

Figure 16 - 5

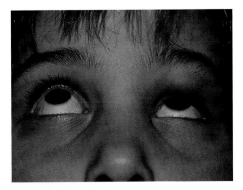

Figure 16 - 6

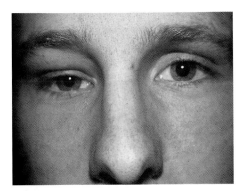

Figure 16 - 7

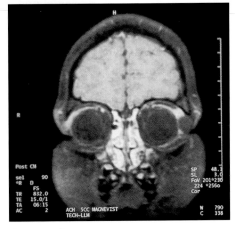

Figure 16 - 8

Figures 16-5 to 16-8 *The clinical appearance and the CT scan of a typical dermoid cyst. The tumor, seen in the middle of the upper orbit (Fig. 16-5), is causing a limitation of upgaze of the left eye (Fig. 16-6). Figure 16-7 shows a large orbital dermoid causing fullness of the upper lid. Figure 16-8 shows a CT scan appearance of an orbital dermoid in the left lateral orbit.*

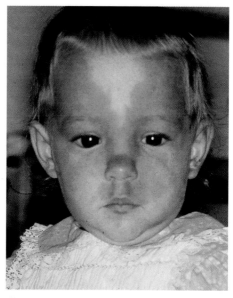

Figure 16 - 9

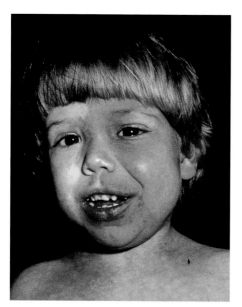

Figure 16 - 10

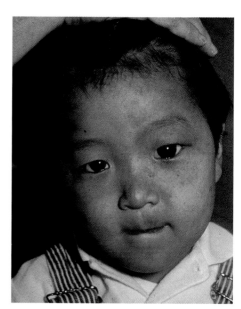

Figure 16 - 11

Figures 16-9 to 16-11   *The appearance of a "flat" nevus flamus type capillary dilation and proliferation which is often associated with Sturge-Weber syndrome. The eyes of these children are at increased risk for glaucoma and choroidal hemagioma, especially when the lesion involves the upper lid.*

OPHTHALMIC DISEASE IN TODDLERS

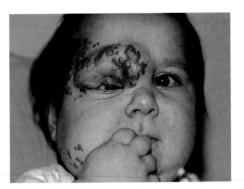

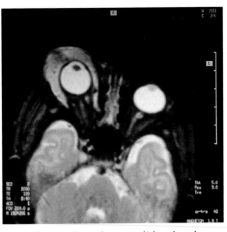

Figures 16-12 and 16-13 *A hemangioma such as this one affecting the right upper lid and scalp (Fig. 16-12) also has diffuse orbital involvement seen in the CT scan of this patient (Fig. 16-13).*

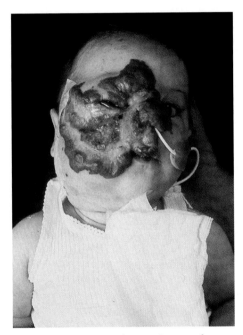

Figure 16-14 *A severe hemangioma such as this is often associated with extensive cranial, facial, and neck involvement, leading to severe disruptions in vision and cognitive and motor development and airway obstruction.*

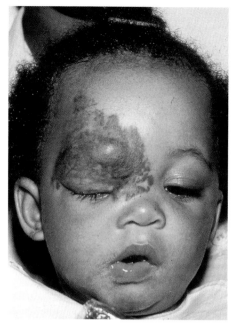

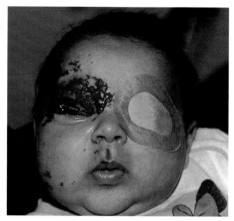

Figures 16-15 and 16-16 *When hemangiomas cause ptosis of the upper lid (Figs. 16-15 and 16-16), they need reduction treatment and occlusion of the sound eye (Fig. 13-1, Chap. 13) to treat the induced deprivation amblyopia.*

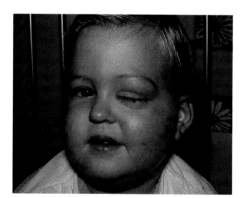

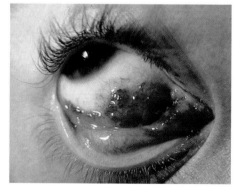

Figures 16-17 and 16-18 *This child has upper lid swelling indicative of an orbital lymphangioma (Fig. 16-17). The diagnosis of this tumor can be made upon examination of the conjunctival surface, where the tumor may be visible (Fig. 16-18).*

OPHTHALMIC DISEASE IN TODDLERS

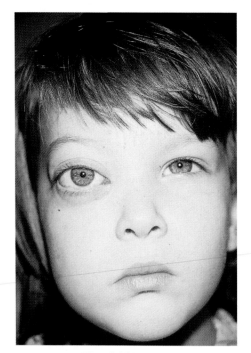

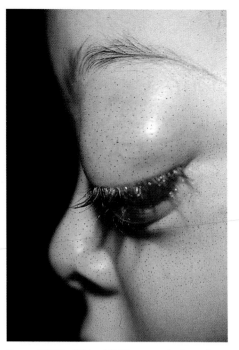

Figure 16-19 *This child has severe proptosis of the globe indicative of an orbital tumor within the muscle cone, a symptom that can be consistent with many primary and metastatic tumors. This was an optic nerve glioma.*

Figure 16-20 *This child has proptosis and lid swelling indicative of an orbital tumor. This symptom can be consistent with many primary and metastatic tumors. This was a rhabdomyosarcoma.*

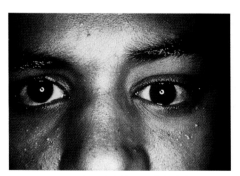

Figure 16-21 *This child has subtle left-eye proptosis and limitation of vertical gaze due to leukemic orbital infiltration.*

SELECTED REFERENCES

Barnes PD et al: Pediatric orbital and visual pathway lesions. *Neuroimaging Clin North Am* 6(1):179–198, 1996.

Campbell A: 2. Tumors of the eye and orbit in childhood. *Nurs Mirror Midwives J* 134(20):26–29, 1972.

Char DH: Management of orbital tumors. *Mayo Clin Proc* 68(11):1081–1096, 1993.

Shields CL, Shields JA, Peggs M: Tumors metastatic to the orbit. *Ophthalmol Plast Reconstr Surg* 4(2):73–80, 1988.

Shields JA, Augsburger JJ, Donoso LA: Orbital dermoid cyst of conjunctival origin. *Am J Ophthalmol* 101(6):726–729, 1986.

Shields JA, Shields CL: Ocular tumors of childhood. *Pediatr Clin North Am* 40(4):805–826, 1993.

Singh AD et al: Primitive neuroectodermal tumor of the orbit. *Arch Ophthalmol* 112(2): 217–221, 1994.

Sykora KW et al: Ophthalmic neoplasms in infancy and childhood. *Pediatrician* 17(3): 163–172, 1990.

INTRAOCULAR AND OCULAR SURFACE TUMORS

JAMES J. AUGSBERGER

Pediatric intraocular tumors constitute a spectrum of malignant and benign neoplasms, hamartomas, and choristomas of the retina, choroid, ciliary body, iris, and optic disc that occur in infants and/or children. Pediatric ocular surface tumors constitute a more limited spectrum of mostly benign neoplasms, hamartomas, and choristomas that occur in infants and/or children.

RETINOBLASTOMA

DEFINITION OF TERMS

Retinoblastoma is a primary intraocular malignant neoplasm that arises from immature retinal cells (retinoblasts) in infants and children. It has a cumulative lifetime incidence of approximately 1 in 15,000 to 1 in 18,000 individuals, almost all of whom are affected prior to the age of 6 years. The average age at diagnosis in most published series is between 12 and 18 months. Untreated, retinoblastoma typically destroys the affected eye within several months to years, extends out of the eye via the optic nerve or scleral vascular or neural foramina, produces massive fungating proptosis, invades the central nervous system, metastasizes widely, and ultimately kills the affected child. At a cellular level, retinoblastoma is a consequence of loss or inactivation of both alleles of a DNA segment (Rb gene) on the long arm of chromosome 13 (locus 13q14). This genetic abnormality results in inability to produce a protein that regulates the cell cycle and normally limits cellular proliferation. Retinoblastoma is a monocular, unifocal disease in about 70% of affected children, but it is a binocular and/or multifocal disease in

about 30%. Approximately 7% to 10% of children with newly diagnosed retinoblastoma have an affected parent or sibling. These children, plus virtually all those with binocular and/or multifocal monocular retinoblastoma and about 10% to 12% of those with no family history of retinoblastoma and unifocal, monocular disease have the hereditary form of retinoblastoma, which is transmitted as an autosomal dominant trait with approximately 90% to 95% penetrance (Figs. 17-1–17-9)

CLINICAL FEATURES

1. Leukokoria (white pupillary reflection)—Present at presentation in about 90% to 95% of patients.
2. Strabismus—Second most common presenting manifestation of retinoblastoma.
3. Rubeosis iridis—Iris neovascularization develops in response to intraocular tumor in large proportion of advanced intraocular cases; sometimes results in spontaneous hyphema, frequently associated with secondary glaucoma.
4. Discrete intraretinal white tumors—Usually with prominent network of fine-caliber intralesional blood vessels plus dilated tortuous feeder and drainer retinal blood vessels.
5. Exophytic growth pattern—Opaque white retinal tumor grows preferentially toward the choroid and sclera, resulting in nonrhegmatogenous retinal detachment; prominent feeder and drainer retinal blood vessels are usually evident.
6. Endophytic growth pattern—Opaque white retinal tumor grows preferentially through internal limiting membrane into the vitre-

ous, resulting in finely dispersed tumor cells and aggregated tumor cell clumps (vitreous seeds) in vitreous; primary tumor appears fluffy white without obvious intralesional or feeder and drainer blood vessels.

7. Multiple hyperreflective intralesional foci within soft-tissue intraocular mass on B-scan ultrasonography—Such foci are attributable to intralesional calcification; such foci are present in about 95% of larger retinoblastoma tumors.
8. Extensive intralesional calcification demonstrable by CT scanning—This feature is also evident in about 95% of larger retinoblastoma tumors.
9. Trilateral retinoblastoma—The occurrence of bilateral retinoblastoma and an independent primitive neuroectodermal tumor (pineoblastoma or ectopic intracranial retinoblastoma) in the sellar, parasellar, or suprasellar region of brain.

DIFFERENTIAL DIAGNOSIS

1. Differential diagnosis of discrete intraretinal retinoblastoma
   a. Astrocytic hamartoma of retina
   b. Intraocular *Toxocara canis* granuloma
   c. Medulloepithelioma
   d. Combined hamartoma of retina
   e. Von Hippel tumor
2. Differential diagnosis of advanced exophytic retinoblastoma
   a. Coats' disease
   b. Persistent hyperplastic primary vitreous
   c. Retrolental fibroplasia
      (i) Retinopathy of prematurity
      (ii) Familial exudative vitreoretinopathy
      (iii) Incontinentia pigmenti retinopathy
   d. Retinal dysplasia
      (i) Norrie's disease
      (ii) Chromosome 18 deletion
      (iii) Chromosome 13 deletion
3. Differential diagnosis of advanced endophytic retinoblastoma
   a. Pars planitis (intermediate uveitis)
   b. Endophthalmitic ocular toxocariasis
   c. Leukemic infiltration of retina and vitreous

WORKUP

1. Family history for retinoblastoma, enucleation or irradiation of one or both eyes in childhood, or unexplained vision loss since childhood
2. CT scan of eyes and orbits
3. MRI of orbits and brain
4. Lumbar puncture for cerebrospinal fluid cytology (advanced cases)
5. Bone marrow aspiration or biopsy for cytology (advanced cases)
6. Molecular genetic analysis of fresh tumor (enucleated cases) (optional)
7. Familial genetic counseling

TREATMENTS

1. Enucleation
2. Chemotherapy
3. External beam radiation therapy
4. Plaque radiation therapy
5. Laser therapy or photocoagulation
6. Cryotherapy

MEDULLOEPITHELIOMA

DEFINITION OF TERMS

Medulloepithelioma is a rare primary intraocular neoplasm of unknown cause that arises from primitive neuroectodermal cells of the developing optic cup. It usually arises from the neural epithelial layers of the ciliary body. The average age at detection is typically 2 to 3 years. Boys and girls are affected with equal frequency. There is no recognized hereditary tendency for this tumor. Some medulloepitheliomas exhibit local growth but no invasive features and are categorized as benign histopathologically. Others exhibit aggressive local invasiveness and are classified as malignant histopathologically. Most medulloepitheliomas, even those classified as malignant, have a limited capacity to metastasize. Some tumors exhibit foci of differentiation into tissues such as cartilage, smooth or striated muscle, or dermal appendages. Tumors containing such tissues are referred to as teratoid medulloepitheliomas. Ones without such tissues are termed nonteratoid medulloepitheliomas (Figs. 17-10–17-12).

CLINICAL FEATURES

1. Iris tumor (amelanotic, usually dull pink to tan) with or without obvious intralesional cysts
2. White mass in ciliary body, with or without intralesional cysts
3. Rubeosis iridis in absence of obvious advanced intraocular retinoblastoma or lesion consistent with juvenile xanthogranuloma

DIFFERENTIAL DIAGNOSIS

1. Retinoblastoma
2. Juvenile xanthogranuloma
3. Lacrimal gland choristoma of iris
4. Glioneuroma (brain choristoma) of iris
5. Peripheral *T. canis* granuloma
6. Leukemic intraocular infiltration

WORKUP

1. General physical examination to rule out juvenile xanthogranulomatosis
2. Complete blood count (CBC) with differential to rule out leukemia
3. CT scan of eyes and orbits to better define and characterize tumor
4. Examination of eyes under anesthesia to assess full extent of lesion and detect subtle associated abnormalities

TREATMENTS

1. Enucleation
2. Excision of well-defined lesions by irido-cyclectomy or cyclectomy

INTRAOCULAR LEUKEMIC INFILTRATES

DEFINITION OF TERMS

Leukemia is a term referring to a broad spectrum of hematologic malignancies. Each is characterized by abnormal leukocytic development and maturation in the bone marrow and high numbers of neoplastic leukocytes in the circulating blood. Most forms of leukemia are referred to by a two-part term that includes a root indicating the predominant leukocytic cell line (e.g., myelo-, lympho-, mono-, eosino-, baso-) and a suffix indicating the degree of anaplasia of the abnormal leukocytes in the circulating blood (e.g., -cytic, -blastic). For example, lymphoblastic and myelocytic are recognized forms of leukemia. All leukemias share the potential to replace normal bone marrow with neoplastic cells, thereby limiting the production of normal leukocytes and erythrocytes and depriving the body of the normal functions provided by those cells. All leukemias can involve the eyes. However, several cross-sectional studies of children with leukemias of various types indicate that the frequency of clinically important intraocular infiltrative lesions is extremely low. Furthermore, most reported intraocular leukemic infiltrates have occurred in patients experiencing relapse of their disease following initial remission in response to chemotherapy (Figs. 17-13 and 17-14).

CLINICAL FEATURES

1. Retinal hemorrhages scattered throughout the fundus of one or both eyes; usually occur in context of severe anemia and/or thrombocytopenia
2. Dilated tortuous retinal veins in patients with substantially elevated white blood cell counts in circulating blood
3. White retinal leukemic infiltrates in occasional patients with relapsed leukemia
4. Ill-defined choroidal leukemic infiltrates, usually associated with nonrhegmatogenous posterior retinal detachment
5. Optic disc leukemic infiltrates
6. Leukemic vitreous cells
7. Leukemic pseudohypopyon

DIFFERENTIAL DIAGNOSIS

1. Microbial retinitis (e.g., cytomegalovirus retinitis)
2. Nonmicrobial inflammatory retinitis or choroiditis

WORKUP

1. Review history regarding prior diagnosis and treatment of leukemia

2. Complete physical examination to evaluate for petechiae, purpura, splenomegaly, etc.
3. CBC with differential count
4. Bone marrow aspiration or biopsy
5. Lumbar puncture to evaluate cerebrospinal fluid cytology
6. Fine-needle aspiration biopsy of cells from aqueous, vitreous, or retina

TREATMENTS

1. Chemotherapy appropriate to type of leukemia
2. External beam radiation therapy

VON HIPPEL TUMOR (RETINAL CAPILLARY HEMANGIOMA)

DEFINITION OF TERMS

The von Hippel tumor is a benign proliferation of cells derived from neurosensory retina plus a reactive proliferation of endothelial-lined capillaries. The lesions characteristically develop during the second decade of life or later. They can be unifocal or multifocal. Most of the multifocal cases also have binocular involvement. The frequency of such tumors is not known precisely but appears to be in the range of 1 in 25,000 individuals. Almost all persons with multifocal or binocular von Hippel tumors have von Hippel–Lindau (VHL) disease, an autosomal dominant disorder that affects about 1 in 36,000 persons. The disease has been linked to a DNA defect in chromosome 3p25-26. Many, if not most, monocular, unifocal cases, especially those diagnosed initially in patients over the age of 40 years, are sporadic and not associated with the genetic defect and other features of VHL (Figs. 17-15 and 17-16)

CLINICAL FEATURES

1. Red spherical intraretinal lesion
2. Dilated feeder and drainer retinal blood vessels
3. Surrounding intraretinal and subretinal exudates
4. Tractional and/or exudative retinal detachment
5. Associated hemangioblastomas of cerebellum, brainstem and spinal cord, renal cell carcinoma, and/or other features of VHL disease

DIFFERENTIAL DIAGNOSIS

1. Retinoblastoma
2. Astrocytic hamartoma of retina
3. Arteriovenous malformation of retina
4. Hemangiomatous peripheral fundus neovascularization
5. Retinal telangiectasis (Coats' disease)

WORKUP

1. Individuals with family history of VHL
   a. Genetic testing for chromosome 3p25-26 defect
   b. Regular periodic screening of affected individuals
   c. Periodic comprehensive ophthalmoscopy
   d. Periodic MRI of brain and spinal cord
   e. Periodic MRI or CT scan of abdomen
2. Individuals with negative family history of VHL but (a) multifocal and/or binocular von Hippel tumors, (b) diagnosis of von Hippel tumor prior to age 40 years, or (c) both
   a. Same testing as recommended for persons having family history of VHL
3. Individuals with negative family history of VHL having a single von Hippel tumor in one eye diagnosed after the age of 40 years
   a. Consider baseline central nervous system (CNS) and abdominal imaging
   b. Follow patients periodically without systemic testing if baseline studies are negative or systemic testing is declined

TREATMENTS

1. Photocoagulation or laser therapy
2. Cryotherapy
3. Plaque radiation therapy
4. Proton beam irradiation
5. Endoresection of tumor
6. Enucleation

CAVERNOUS HEMANGIOMA OF RETINA

DEFINITION OF TERMS

The cavernous hemangioma of the retina is a benign clustering of thin-walled intraretinal vascular saccules lined by mature endothelial cells. It is essentially a vascular birthmark of the retina.

It usually occurs sporadically as a single lesion in one eye, but it occurs occasionally multifocally and/or bilaterally, sometimes in families with apparent autosomal dominant clustering. Most lesions of this type enlarge minimally if at all throughout life, and malignant transformation is unknown. Larger lesions tend to be detected early in life, whereas smaller lesions are frequently not detected until the second decade of life or later (Figs. 17-17 and 17-18)

CLINICAL FEATURES

1. Dark red intraretinal vascular saccules of various sizes
2. Anomalous retinal vein passing through lesion
3. Superficial retinal gliosis

DIFFERENTIAL DIAGNOSIS

1. Idiopathic retinal telangiectasis (Coats' disease)
2. Perifoveal telangiectasia

WORKUP

1. No workup generally indicated
2. Examine first-degree relatives to look for familial clustering
3. MRI of brain in patients with prominent fundus lesion or familial clustering

TREATMENTS

1. No treatment is usually indicated
2. Cryotherapy
3. Posterior vitrectomy

COMBINED HAMARTOMA OF RETINA

DEFINITION OF TERMS

The combined hamartoma of the retina is a benign retinal mass composed of disorganized sensory retina, secondary reactive intraretinal gliosis, proliferation and intraretinal migration of the underlying retinal pigment epithelium, and abnormally prominent and tortuous intralesional retinal blood vessels. The lesion has no known malignant potential. It is usually a unilateral, uni-

focal lesion. It is believed to be a congenital abnormality in most if not all cases. Many patients with such lesions have subsequently been noted to have neurofibromatosis (NF), especially NF-2. Combined hamartomas of the retina usually arise in a juxtapapillary or circumpapillary location, but similar-appearing lesions have occasionally been detected in the peripheral fundus. The precise frequency of this lesion is unknown but appears to be in the range of 1 in 50,000 to 1 in 100,000 persons (Fig. 17-19).

CLINICAL FEATURES

1. Localized juxtapapillary or circumpapillary lesion with intraretinal and preretinal gliosis, underlying proliferation and intraretinal migration of retinal pigment epithelial cells, and tortuous and angulated retinal blood vessels within lesion
2. Amblyopia—Occurs if lesion involves macula

DIFFERENTIAL DIAGNOSIS

1. Choroidal melanoma
2. Retinoblastoma
3. Astrocytic hamartoma of retina
4. Medulloepithelioma
5. Reactive vitreoretinal fibrosis

WORKUP

1. Comprehensive physical examination to evaluate for NF-2
2. MRI of brain to evaluate for bilateral acoustic neuromas

TREATMENTS

1. No treatment is generally recommended.
2. Posterior vitrectomy with membrane peeling has been attempted but is generally not beneficial.

DIFFUSE AND CIRCUMSCRIBED CHOROIDAL HEMANGIOMAS

DEFINITION OF TERMS

A choroidal hemangioma is a benign neoplasm or hamartoma composed of mature blood vessels ranging from capillaries to large cavernous channels. Two varieties of choroidal hemangioma are recognized. The diffuse choroidal hemangioma is a generalized thickening of the choroid by capillary and cavernous blood vessels, sometimes with localized nodular accentuation posteriorly. The choroidal thickening tends to be most pronounced in the macular and circumpapillary regions and least pronounced in the periphery. The diffuse choroidal hemangioma is characteristically associated with an ipsilateral facial nevus flammeus and can be associated with ipsilateral leptomeningeal hemangiomatosis and other vascular malformations. The circumscribed choroidal hemangioma is a localized but often poorly defined nodular vascular tumor of the posterior choroid. It almost always arises near the optic disc and/or fovea. Both forms of choroidal hemangioma can enlarge slowly, but malignant transformation has never been reported. The precise frequency of such lesions is unknown. Virtually all cir-cumscribed choroidal hemangiomas occur unilaterally, but occasional diffuse choroidal hemangiomas occur bilaterally, usually in association with facial nevus flammeus involving both sides of the face (Figs. 17-20–17-25).

CLINICAL FEATURES

1. Diffuse choroidal hemangioma
   a. Facial nevus flammeus
   b. Asymmetric pupillary red reflex
   c. Asymmetric fundus features
2. Circumscribed choroidal hemangioma
   a. Localized but ill-defined reddish orange choroidal lesion
   b. Cystic retinal degeneration overlying choroidal lesion
   c. White fibrous metaplasia of retinal pigment epithelium overlying lesion
   d. Nonrhegmatogenous retinal detachment

DIFFERENTIAL DIAGNOSIS

1. Differential diagnosis of diffuse choroidal hemangioma
2. Differential diagnosis of circumscribed choroidal hemangioma
   a. Amelanotic choroidal nevus versus melanoma

WORKUP

1. Workup for diffuse choroidal hemangioma
   a. Comprehensive ophthalmic glaucoma evaluation and follow-up
   b. Periodic fundus examination to evaluate for exudative retinal detachment
   c. CT scan or MRI of brain to evaluate for ipsilateral meningeal hemangiomatosis
2. Workup for circumscribed choroidal hemangioma
   a. ICG angiogram of fundus lesions with late images

TREATMENTS

1. Treatments for diffuse choroidal hemangiomas
   a. External beam radiation therapy
2. Treatments for circumscribed choroidal hemangiomas
   a. Plaque radiation therapy
   b. External beam radiation therapy
   c. Laser therapy or photocoagulation

ASTROCYTIC HAMARTOMA OF RETINA

DEFINITION OF TERMS

The astrocytic hamartoma of the retina is a benign, relatively well-differentiated neoplasm that arises from astrocytes in the neurosensory retina. Rarely congenital, it is most frequently diagnosed in older children, adolescents, and young adults. Lesions that grow more rapidly and achieve a relatively larger size tend to be detected at an earlier patient age than are smaller, slowly growing lesions. It occurs in a monocular, unifocal, usually nonsyndromic form and in a binocular and/or multifocal, usually syndromic form associated with other features of tuberous sclerosis. It is inherited as an autosomal dominant disorder with variable expressivity and penetrance and has been associated with small deletions of a gene on the short arm of chromosome 9 and occasionally on chromosome 3 (Figs. 17-26 and 17-27).

CLINICAL FEATURES

1. Translucent retinal patches—Early lesions frequently appear as ill-defined translucent superficial retinal patches.
2. Opaque white retinal lesions—More advanced lesions appear better defined and opaque white; typical lesions arise from inner retinal layers and overlie normal retinal blood vessels.
3. Dense lesions with intralesional calcification—Advanced lesions occasionally become dense and calcified; such lesions have been said to resemble rock candy.
4. Multifocal retinal lesions—Multiple lesions in one eye and/or bilateral retinal lesions develop in many patients with tuberous sclerosis; individual lesions can exhibit the entire spectrum described above.
5. Adenoma sebaceum of face and other clinical features of tuberous sclerosis.

DIFFERENTIAL DIAGNOSIS

1. Retinoblastoma
2. Retinal *T. canis* granuloma

WORKUP

1. Comprehensive physical examination to evaluate for extraophthalmic features of tuberous sclerosis
   a. Ash leaf spots of skin
   b. Adenoma sebaceum of facial skin
   c. Shagreen patches of skin
   d. Subungual or periungual fibromas
2. CT scan or MRI of brain, chest, abdomen to evaluate for other lesions of tuberous sclerosis
   a. Cysts of liver, pancreas, lungs
   b. Benign tumors of kidney
   c. Cardiac rhabdomyomas
3. Examination of close relatives

TREATMENTS

1. No treatment is usually indicated.
2. Enucleation—Limited to advanced cases causing profound loss of vision and/or blind, painful eye and to some lesions that cannot reliably be differentiated from retinoblastoma.

CHOROIDAL OSTEOMA

DEFINITION OF TERMS

The choroidal osteoma is a benign neoplasm or choristoma composed of mature bone. The precise frequency of such tumors is unknown, but it appears to be <1 in 100,000 individuals. The typical patient with a choroidal osteoma is between 15 and 25 years of age at the time of initial lesion detection. Most lesions of this type (>90%) occur in females. Approximately 20% of affected persons develop bilateral lesions. Almost all such lesions arise in the juxtapapillary choroid and eventually extend partially or completely around the optic disc. Slow lesion enlargement occurs over the course of years, but malignant transformation has not been reported. No cause is generally evident. Serum calcium, phosphorus, and parathyroid hormone levels are generally within normal limits in affected patients (Figs. 17-28–17-30).

CLINICAL FEATURES

1. Golden, yellow-white, or orange color
2. Juxtapapillary or circumpapillary lesion location
3. Well-defined, smoothly curved margins
4. Disruption of macular retina and occasional overlying choroidal neovascularization
5. Dense, highly reflective plate corresponding to lesion on B-scan ultrasonography
6. Bone-dense platelike lesion conforming to posterior eye wall on CT scan

DIFFERENTIAL DIAGNOSIS

1. Idiopathic sclerochoroidal calcification
2. Degenerative chorioretinal calcification
3. Choroidal cartilaginous choristoma in Aicardi's syndrome
4. Circumscribed choroidal hemangioma

WORKUP

1. Comprehensive ophthalmoscopy
2. B-scan ophthalmic ultrasonography
3. CT scan of eyes and orbits
4. Fluorescein angiography if choroidal neovascularization is suspected

TREATMENTS

1. No treatment is generally indicated
2. Focal photocoagulation for extrafoveal choroidal neovascularization

CONJUNCTIVAL NEVUS

DEFINITION OF TERMS

The conjunctival nevus is a benign melanocytic tumor that arises from neural crest–derived melanocytes within the basal layers of the conjunctival epithelium or the conjunctival substantia propria. The nevus is rarely evident at birth, but typically becomes apparent later in the first decade or early in the second decade of life. Hormonal factors related to puberty may influence development of such lesions. Histopathologically, the conjunctival nevus consists of atypical, prominent melanocytes with benign nuclear and nucleolar characteristics within (1) the basal epithelium only, (2) both the basal epithelium and superficial adjacent substantia propria (junctional), or (3) the substantia propria only (subepithelial). These lesions have extremely low malignant potential but are usually excised because malignant melanoma of the conjunctiva cannot be excluded (Figs. 17-31–17-33).

CLINICAL FEATURES

1. Focal melanotic conjunctival lesions
2. Focal amelanotic conjunctival lesions
3. Diffuse conjunctival lesions
4. Cystic conjunctival lesions

DIFFERENTIAL DIAGNOSIS

1. Malignant melanoma of conjunctiva
2. Ocular melanocytosis
3. Conjunctival foreign body
4. Conjunctival argyrosis
5. Ocular ochronosis
6. Juvenile xanthogranuloma of conjunctiva

WORKUP

1. Comprehensive ophthalmic physical examination

TREATMENTS

1. Observation
2. Excision

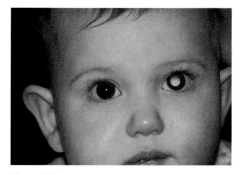

Figure 17-1

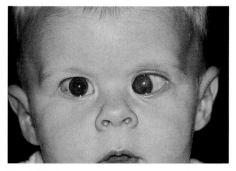

Figure 17-2

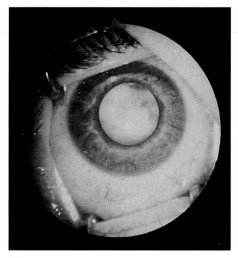

Figure 17-3

Figures 17-1 to 17-3 *Retinoblastoma often causes leukokoria (Fig. 17-1, left eye) and strabismus (left esotropia, Fig. 17-2). The child in Fig. 17-2 also has a cloudy cornea and enlarged corneal diameter on the left due to tumor-related neovascular glaucoma. Figure 17-3 shows rubeosis iridis and leukokoria associated with advanced intraocular retinoblastoma.*

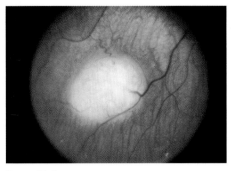

Figure 17-4

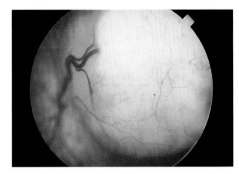

Figure 17-5

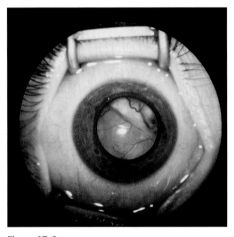

Figure 17-6

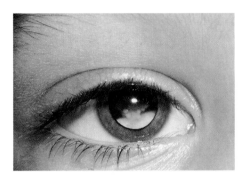

Figure 17-7

Figures 17-4 to 17-7 *These photographs of intraocular retinoblastoma show the tumor as opaque, white, and having a fine network of superficial intralesional blood vessels (Fig. 17-4). Figure 17-5 shows a larger tumor than that shown in Fig. 17-4, and it exhibits prominent retinal feeder and drainer blood vessels. Figure 17-6 shows an exophytic growth pattern of advanced intraocular retinoblastoma. Characteristic features include opaque white subretinal tumor with dilated retinal blood vessels on its surface and an associated nonrhegmatogenous retinal detachment. Figure 17-7 shows an endophytic growth pattern of advanced intraocular retinoblastoma. Characteristic features include fluffy white tumor mass without evident blood vessels and dispersed intravitreal tumor cell clumps (tumor seeds).*

OPHTHALMIC DISEASE IN TODDLERS

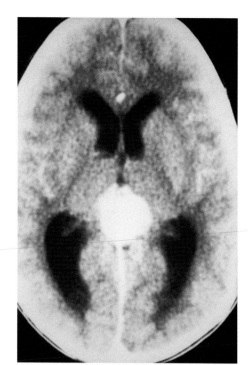

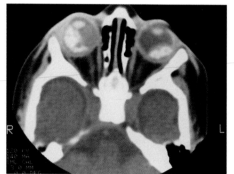

Figures 17-8 and 17-9 *CT scans of a bilateral retinoblastoma, demonstrating near bone density of retinal tumors in each eye (Fig. 17-8), and an ectopic intracranial retinoblastoma in the brain of a child with bilateral retinoblastoma, referred to as trilateral retinoblastoma (Fig. 17-9).*

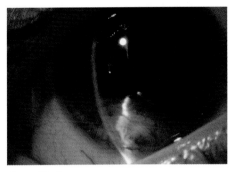

Figure 17-10

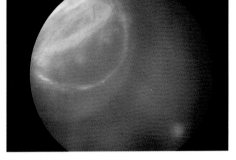

Figure 17-11

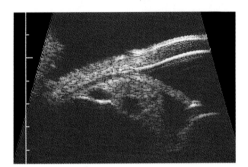

Figure 17-12

Figures 17-10 to 17-12 *Intraocular medullo-epithelioma presenting as an iris mass (Fig. 17-10) and as a white ciliary body mass with prominent cyst projecting into vitreous (Fig. 17-11). Figure 17-12 shows a high-frequency (20-MHz) B-scan ultrasound image of medulloepithelioma of ciliary body with prominent cysts within solid soft-tissue mass.*

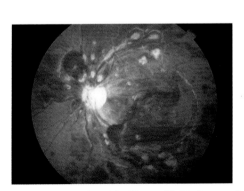

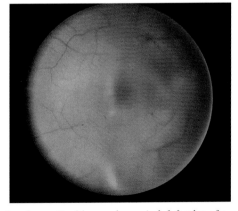

Figures 17-13 and 17-14 *Figure 17-13 shows retinal and preretinal hemorrhages in left fundus of a 13-year-old girl with acute lymphocytic leukemia (courtesy of Dr. George Kranias). Figure 17-14 shows leukemic cells in vitreous of an adolescent boy with relapsed acute lymphocytic leukemia.*

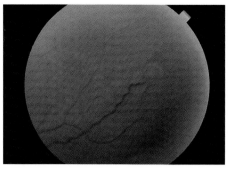
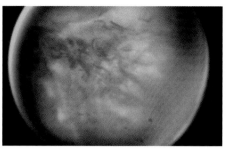

Figures 17-15 and 17-16   *A small peripheral von Hippel tumor appearing as a spherical red intraretinal lesion (Fig. 17-15). Figure 17-16 shows a large von Hippel tumor and the retina highly detached, with tractional and exudative components. Dilated, tortuous retinal feeder and drainer blood vessels are apparent (Fig. 17-16).*

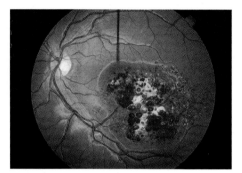
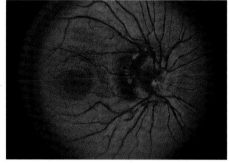

Figures 17-17 and 17-18   *Typical cavernous hemangiomas of the retina. The lesion in Fig. 17-17 consists of dark red vascular saccules of various sizes accompanied by white superficial retinal gliosis, whereas Fig. 17-18 shows a lesion involving the optic disc. Vascular saccules that make up the lesion are apparent.*

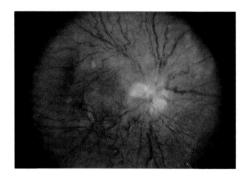

Figure 17-19   *A combined hamartoma of the retina in a 2-year-old boy who was later found to have neurofibromatosis type 2. Components of the lesion include gliotic thickening of retina, proliferation and intraretinal migration of the underlying retinal pigment epithelium, and abnormal vascular prominence and tortuosity within the lesion.*

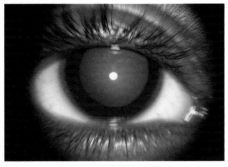

Figure 17-20

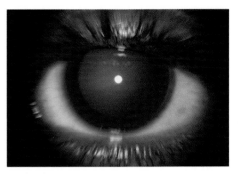

Figure 17-21

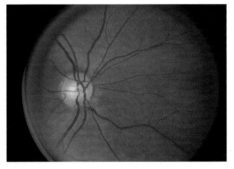

Figure 17-22

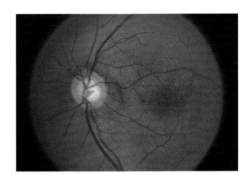

Figure 17-23

Figures 17-20 to 17-23 *The pupillary red reflexes in right eye (Fig. 17-20) and left eye (Fig. 17-21) of a patient with right-sided facial nevus flammeus and ipsilateral diffuse choroidal hemangioma. Note the more saturated red color of pupillary light reflex from right eye. Figures 17-22 and 17-23 show the asymmetric fundus appearance of right eye (Fig. 17-22) and left eye (Fig. 17-23) of a patient with diffuse choroidal hemangioma of the left eye. Note the more saturated red appearance of left fundus, thickening of the choroid around the optic disc, resulting in a deep disc cup in the left eye, and obscuration of the normal large choroidal blood vessels that are evident in the right fundus nasal to the optic disc.*

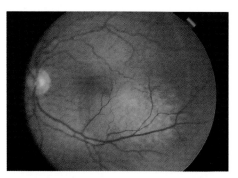
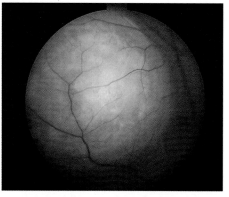

Figures 17-24 and 17-25 *A circumscribed choroidal hemangioma (Fig. 17-24) and a large circumscribed choroidal hemangioma with overlying white fibrous metaplasia of retinal pigment epithelium (Fig. 17-25).*

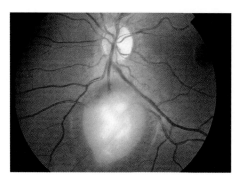
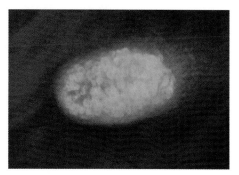

Figures 17-26 and 17-27 *Astrocytic hamartomas of retina. Figure 17-26 shows a lesion below the optic disc appearing as a focal opaque white retinal lesion, and Fig. 17-27 shows a lesion appearing as a dense, calcified, white retinal tumor arising from the inner retina.*

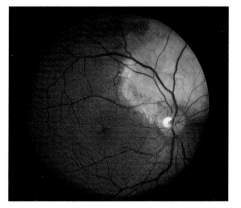

Figure 17-28

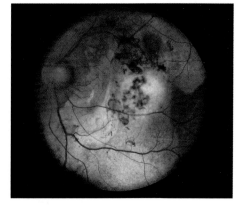

Figure 17-29

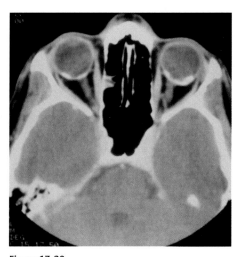

Figure 17-30

Figures 17-28 to 17-30 *This choroidal osteoma appears as a well-defined yellowish-white superior juxtapapillary lesion in right eye (Fig. 17-28). Figure 17-29 shows a choroidal osteoma in left eye of same patient that is substantially larger than the lesion in the right fundus; however, it has a similar color and similarly well-defined margins. The sensory retina and retinal pigment epithelium in the macula are severely disrupted. Figure 17-30 shows a CT scan (axial image) of orbits in a patient with bilateral choroidal osteoma. Note bone-dense plates corresponding to the posterior choroidal lesion in each eye.*

OPHTHALMIC DISEASE IN TODDLERS

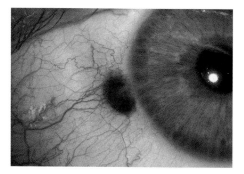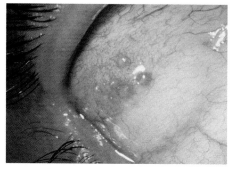

Figures 17-31 and 17-32 *A well-defined dark brown limbal conjunctival nevus in a 12-year-old boy (Fig. 17-31) and a partially cystic melanotic limbal conjunctival nevus (Fig. 17-32).*

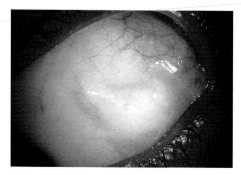

Figure 17-33 *An epibulbar osseous choristoma in the superotemporal bulbar region of the left eye.*

SELECTED REFERENCES

Augsburger JJ, Shields JA, Moffat KP: Circumscribed choroidal hemangiomas: long term visual prognosis. *Retina* 1:56–61, 1981.

Colvard DM, Robertson DM, Trautman JC: Cavernous hemangioma of the retina. *Arch Ophthalmol* 96:2042–2044, 1978.

Daily EG, Lubowitz RM. Dermoids of the limbus and cornea. *Am J Ophthalmol* 53:661–665, 1962.

Dreizen NG et al: Epibulbar osseous choristoma. *J Pediatr Ophthalmol Strabismus* 20:247–249, 1983.

Eng C et al: Mortality from second tumors amoung long-term survivors of retinoblastoma. *J Natl Cancer Inst* 85:1121–1128, 1993.

Folberg R et al: Benign conjunctival melanocytic lesions. Clinicopathologic features. *Ophthalmology* 96:436–461, 1989.

Guyer DR et al: Leukemic retinopathy. Relationship between fundus lesions and hematologic parameters at diagnosis. *Ophthalmology* 96:860–864, 1989.

Leonardy NJ et al: Analysis of 135 autopsy eyes for ocular involvement in leukemia. *Am J Ophthalmol* 109:436–444, 1990.

McDonnell JM et al: Conjunctival melanocytic lesions in children. *Ophthalmology* 96:986–993, 1989.

Maher ER, Kaelin WG: Von Hippel–Lindau disease. *Medicine* 76:381–391, 1997.

Meyers SM et al: Retinal changes associated with neurofibromatosis 2. *Trans Am Ophthalmol Soc* 93:245–252, 1995.

Nyboer JH, Robertson DM, Gomez MR: Retinal lesions in tuberous sclerosis. *Arch Ophthalmol* 94:1277–1280, 1976.

Schachat AP et al: Combined hamartomas of the retina and retinal pigment epithelium. *Ophthalmology* 91:1609–1615, 1984.

Shields CL, Shields JA, Augsburger JJ: Choroidal osteoma. *Surv Ophthalmol* 33:17–27, 1988.

Shields JA et al: Congenital neoplasms of the nonpigmented ciliary epithelium (medulloepithelioma). *Ophthalmology* 103:1998–2006, 1996.

Smith BJ, O'Brien JM: The genetics of retinoblastoma and current diagnostic testing. *J Pediatr Ophthalmol Strabismus* 33:120–123, 1996.

Webster AR, Maher ER, Moore AT: Clinical characterization of ocular angiomatosis in von Hippel–Lindau disease and correlation with germline mutation. *Arch Ophthalmol* 117:371–378, 1999.

Witschel H, Font RL: Hemangioma of the choroid. A clinicopathologic study of 71 cases and a review of the literature. *Surv Ophthalmol* 20:415–431, 1976.

PART IV

OPHTHALMIC DISEASE IN SCHOOL-AGE CHILDREN

UVEITIS

CHAUNDRA ROY
and ROBERT B. NUSSENBLATT

DEFINITION OF TERMS

Uveitis refers to inflammation of the uveal tract. The uveal tract comprises the iris, ciliary body, and choroid. Inflammation of adjacent structures such as the retina, known as retinitis, and the sclera, known as scleritis, are often associated with uveitis. Uveitis can result in significant morbidity and visual handicap.

The classification of uveitis by anatomic localization is critical for communicating with other physicians and for generating a useful differential diagnosis. The American Uveitis Society has agreed on four subcategories of uveitis based upon location; they are anterior uveitis, intermediate uveitis, posterior uveitis, and panuveitis. *Anterior uveitis* (*iritis* and *iridocyclitis*) refers to inflammation of the iris and/or ciliary body. *Intermediate uveitis* refers to inflammation of the posterior ciliary body, the pars plana (*pars planitis*) and/or peripheral retina. *Posterior uveitis* refers to inflammation of the choroid (*choroiditis*) or overlying retina (*retinitis*). *Retinal vasculitis* describes a predominant finding of retinal vascular inflammation. The term *vitritis* refers to the presence of inflammatory cells in the vitreous and is classified as intermediate or posterior uveitis depending on the confluence of accompanying signs. *Panuveitis* refers to inflammation involving the entire uveal tract.

COMPLICATIONS OF UVEITIS

1. Decreased vision or blindness
2. Cataract (Fig. 18-1)
3. Glaucoma
4. Cystoid macular edema
5. Band keratopathy
6. Retinal detachment
7. Sensory strabismus
8. Amblyopia
9. Pain or irritation
10. Altered cosmesis
11. Psychosocial issues associated with loss of vision, frequent doctor's visits, frequent surgeries, and altered appearance
12. Therapy-associated side effects

DIFFERENTIAL DIAGNOSIS

The differential diagnosis varies based upon the type of uveitis. The differential diagnosis may be further stratified into infectious and noninfectious causes of uveitis. The noninfectious causes of uveitis most commonly encountered include those associated with systemic autoimmune diseases. The most common systemic disease associated with uveitis in the pediatric population is juvenile rheumatoid arthritis.

The age of the patient and the presence of associated signs and symptoms help to narrow the differential diagnosis. The differential diagnosis listed below is useful in differentiating the most frequently encountered entities.

1. Anterior uveitis
   a. Infectious: Herpes simplex, herpes zoster virus, Epstein-Barr virus
   b. Noninfectious: Idiopathic, juvenile rheumatoid arthritis (JRA) (Figs. 18-1–18-5), sarcoidosis, HLA B27–associated syndromes (ankylosing spondylitis, inflammatory bowel disease, psoriatic arthritis, Reiter's syndrome), Kowasaki's syndrome, Fuchs' heterochromic iridocyclitis, Posner-Schlossman syndrome, masquerade syndromes (ocular lymphoma), trauma
2. Intermediate uveitis
   a. Infectious: Lyme disease, syphilis
   b. Noninfectious: Idiopathic, sarcoidosis, inflammatory bowel disease, intermediate uveitis of pars planitis subtype

3. Posterior uveitis
   a. Infectious: Toxoplasmosis, toxocariasis, syphilis, tuberculosis, Lyme disease, cytomegalovirus, herpes simplex virus, herpes zoster virus
   b. Noninfectious: Idiopathic, sarcoidosis, Behçet's disease (Figs. 18-8–18-9), Vogt-Koyanagi-Harada syndrome, sympathetic ophthalmia, masquerade syndromes (ocular lymphoma)
4. Panuveitis
   a. Infectious: Syphilis, tuberculosis, toxoplasmosis
   b. Noninfectious: Idiopathic, sarcoidosis, Behçet's disease, Vogt-Koyanagi-Harada syndrome, sympathetic ophthalmia, masquerade syndromes (ocular lymphoma)

WORKUP

The evaluation of a patient with uveitis should vary with the clinical presentation and should be directed toward confirming the most likely diagnosis based upon the clinical assessment. A complete history and physical examination by the primary care provider or appropriate specialist is crucial for generating a differential diagnosis.

1. Complete history and physical
2. Complete ophthalmologic examination
3. Complete blood count and white blood cell (WBC) differential
4. Syphilis serology
5. Chest x-ray
6. Tuberculosis skin testing with anergy testing

TREATMENT

Therapy for uveitis should be based upon the ophthalmic findings and response to therapy. Often the ophthalmologist and primary care physician or pediatric subspecialist work together to follow the patient's systemic status and monitor therapy side effects.

Therapy is typically nonspecific and directed at decreasing local or associated systemic inflammation. Specific antimicrobial therapy may be warranted when an infectious etiology is known or suspected.

1. Topical corticosteroids, e.g., prednisolone acetate 1%
2. Local steroid injections, e.g., into sub-Tenon's capsule or subconjunctival injection of Kenalog 20–40 mg
3. Dilating drops, e.g., tropicamide 1%, atropine 1%, or scopolamine 0.25% once or twice daily; the benefit of using cycloplegic agents is the decreased formation of posterior synechiae, which are adhesions of the iris to the underlying anterior capsule of the lens.
4. Nonsteroidal antiinflammatory agents appear to have a limited role in treating pediatric uveitis.
5. Systemic corticosteroids, e.g., prednisone 0.5–2 mg/kg; patients on systemic steroids need to be carefully monitored by a physician familiar with the side-effect profile.
6. Systemic immunosuppressives should be used only in conjunction with a physician experienced with their use.
7. Preventive medicine
   a. Patients on high-dose corticosteroids or immunotherapy should not receive live-virus vaccines (immunize before therapy if possible).
8. Specific antibiotic therapy
   a. Antiherpetic therapy
   b. Specific antimicrobial agent
9. Surgical therapy
   a. Chelation of band keratopathy
   b. Glaucoma surgery
   c. Cataract surgery
   d. Diagnostic or therapeutic vitrectomy

CONCLUSIONS

Uveitis is a vision-threatening condition. Prompt and aggressive diagnosis and treatment in children can alter the natural history and result in favorable visual outcomes.

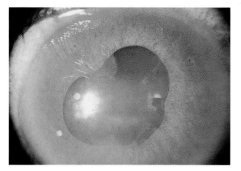

Figure 18-1

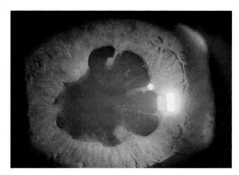

Figure 18-2

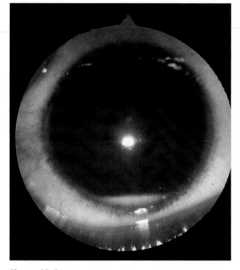

Figure 18-3

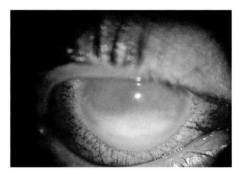

Figure 18-4

Figures 18-1 to 18-4 *Autoimmune inflammation of the anterior uvea (iris and ciliary body) is associated with juvenile rheumatoid arthritis, most commonly present in females with the pauciarticular form with antinuclear antibody (ANA)+, rheumatoid-negative serology. This "clinically silent" inflammation can result in cataract, posterior synechiae, glaucoma, and band keratopathy. Figures 18-1 and 18-2 show the irregular, "fixed" pupils due to adhesions of the iris to the lens (posterior synechiae) resulting from anterior chamber inflammation. Figures 18-3 and 18-4 show the autoimmune accumulation of anterior chamber white cells (hypopyon) due to severe iridocyclitis associated with HLA B27–positive spondyloarthropathies.*

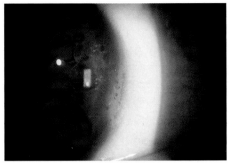

Figure 18-5 *Band keratopathy, a pathologic accumulation of calcium between the corneal epithelium and Bowman's membrane. This finding is common in pediatric patients with chronic ocular inflammation of any etiology. The deposits typically accumulate in the corneal periphery in the region of the interpalpebral fissure. Band keratopathy is frequently asymptomatic, but may result in ocular surface irritation or more rarely may impair vision in advanced cases involving the visual axis.*

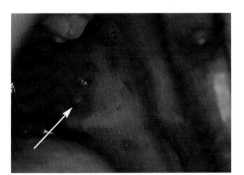

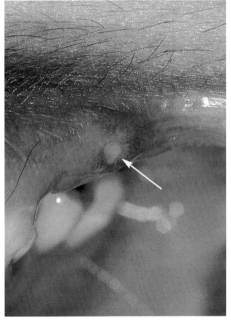

Figures 18-6 and 18-7 *Oral mucosal ulceration in pediatric Behçet's disease (recurrent oral aphthous ulcers, episodic rash, evidence of pathergy, and a history of genital lesions; arrows show ulcers).*

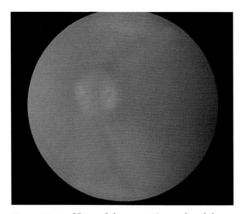

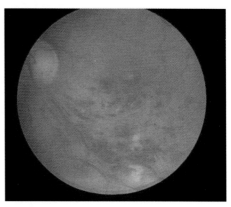

Figure 18-8 *View of the posterior pole of the left eye in a patient with pediatric Behçet's disease showing the hazy media and decreased clarity due to vitritis (vitreous cells and protein exudation).*

Figure 18-9 *High-power view of the left macula at a follow-up visit showing retinal hemorrhages and yellow lipid exudates, sequelae of pediatric Behçet's disease.*

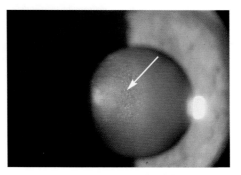

Figure 18-10 *This photograph of the lens shows a posterior subcapsular cataract, also a common sequela of intraocular inflammation and of chronic steroid therapy.*

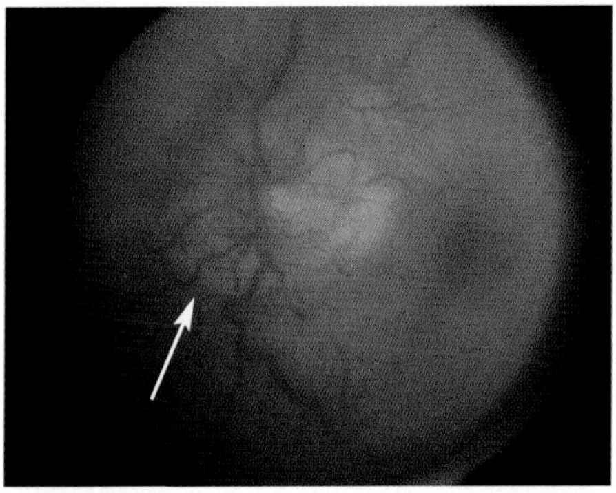

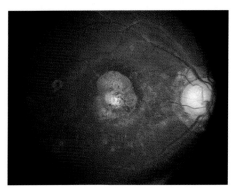

Figure 18-11

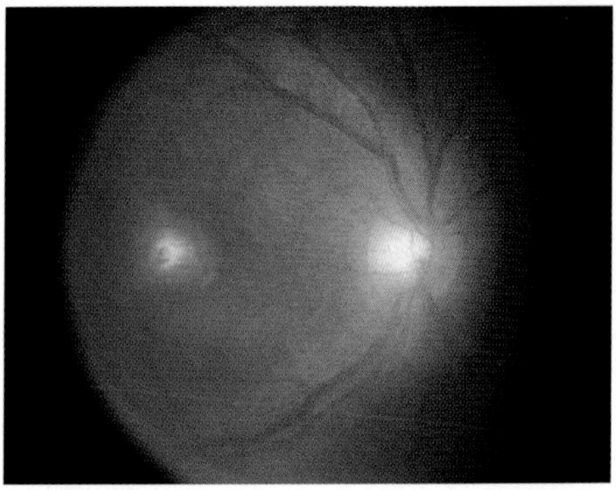

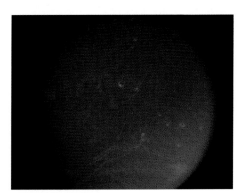

Figure 18-12

Figure 18-13

Figure 18-14

Figures 18-11 to 18-14 *Intraocular complications of pediatric sarcoidosis. Figure 18-11 shows the posterior pole with a circumferential peripapillary granuloma, and Fig. 18-12 shows an early macular granuloma formation. Figure 18-13 shows advanced optic nerve cupping and multiple chorioretinal scars due to secondary glaucoma and past episodes of chorioretinal inflammation. Figure 18-14 shows sheathing of the retinal vessels typical of retinal periphlebitis associated with sarcoidosis.*

OPHTHALMIC DISEASE IN SCHOOL-AGE CHILDREN

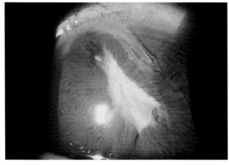

Figure 18-15 *A dense, white, fibrous pupillary membrane that developed postoperatively in a 15-year-old African-American male with chronic idiopathic intermediate uveitis. Uveitis patients present a unique surgical challenge due to their propensity to develop postoperative complications such as increased inflammation, cystoid macular edema, hypotony, and pupillary membrane formation.*

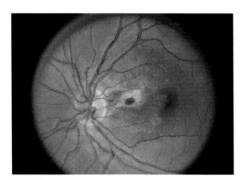

Figure 18-16 *A fibrosed, neovascular granuloma involving the macula from a 16-year-old male with unilateral, idiopathic posterior uveitis.*

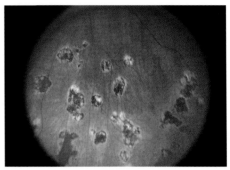

Figure 18-17 *Peripheral chorioretinal scars in the retina that are evidence of a previous multifocal choroiditis of unknown cause.*

SELECTED REFERENCES

Cassidy JT: Medical management of children with juvenile rheumatoid arthritis. *Drugs* 58(5):831–850, 1999.

Hoover DL et al: Pediatric ocular sarcoidosis. *Surv Ophthalmol* 30(4):215–228, 1986.

Nussenblatt R et al: *Uveitis: Fundamentals and Clinical Practice.* St Louis, Mosby-Year Book, 1996.

Pivetti-Pezzi P: Uveitis in children. *Eur J Ophthalmol* 6(3):293–298, 1996.

Rychwalski PJ et al: Asymptomatic uveitis in young people with inflammatory bowel disease. *J Am Assoc Pediatr, Ophthalmol Strabismus* 1(2):111–114, 1997.

Shetty AK, Gedalia A: Sarcoidosis: A pediatric perspective. *Clin Pediatr* 37(12):707–717, 1998.

Singh S et al: Clinico-immunological profile of juvenile rheumatoid arthritis in Chandigarh. *Indian Pediatr* 36(5):449–454, 1999.

NYSTAGMUS AND ANOMALOUS HEAD POSTURES

MITRA MAYBODI

DEFINITION OF TERMS

Anomalous head posture and *torticollis* are the terms used to describe abnormal head positioning. Clinical descriptions include a head or face turn to the right or left, chin up or down, head tilt to right or left, or any combination of these various positions. The earliest age at which head posture may be detected is around 3 months, when the infant gains head control.

Nystagmus is a rhythmic, involuntary oscillation of one or both eyes. Some forms of nystagmus are physiologic, whereas others are pathologic. In evaluating a patient with an anomalous head posture, nystagmus should be considered. The clinical characteristics of nystagmus are usually in the direction of the fast phase and are termed horizontal, vertical, or rotary, or any combination of these. The nystagmus may be conjugate or dysconjugate. The nystagmus may be predominantly pendular or jerky, the former referring to equal-velocity to-and-fro movement of the eyes, and the latter referring to the eyes moving faster in one direction and slower in the other.

DIFFERENTIAL DIAGNOSIS

Anomalous head postures in childhood are mostly the result of abnormalities of the

1. Central nervous system
2. Ocular motor system, including
   a. Strabismus (see Chaps. 7 and 13)
   b. Nystagmus (see below)
   c. Unusual or high refractive errors (hyperopia and astigmatism)
   d. Lid anomalies—most often creating a chin-up position to view below ptotic eyelid(s)

3. Neck musculature anomalies
4. A distant fourth diagnosis is Sandifer syndrome, a congenital condition characterized by gastroesophageal reflux and anomalous head posture
5. Hemianopia with visual field loss

The physiologic forms of nystagmus are

1. Endpoint nystagmus—A jerk nystagmus of fine amplitude that occurs on extreme lateral gaze.
2. Vestibular nystagmus—A jerk nystagmus that can be evoked by altering the equilibrium of the endolymph in the semicircular canals.
3. Optokinetic nystagmus—An induced jerk nystagmus elicited by moving repetitive visual stimuli across the visual field, for example, by looking through the window of a moving train.
4. Voluntary nystagmus—Usually very rapid and horizontal, often associated with convergence of the eyes and pupillary constriction; rarely able to be sustained for more than 30 s at a time.

The types of nystagmus associated with neurologic disorders are

1. Convergence-retraction nystagmus—Cocontraction of all the extraocular muscles with convergence on attempted upward gaze, suggesting a midbrain disorder; consider congenital aqueductal stenosis in infants and pinealoma or hydrocephalus in children.
2. Seesaw nystagmus—A torsional and pendular oscillation of both eyes in which one eye rises and intorts while the other falls and extorts. It may be congenital, but the majority of patients have large parasellar tumors expanding within the third ventri-

cle, and it may be associated with bitemporal hemianopia.

3. Periodic alternating nystagmus—A horizontal jerk nystagmus in which the direction of the jerk, or fast phase, alternates every 1 to 2 min. It is associated with cerebellar or caudal medullary disorders.

4. Downbeat nystagmus—Rapid downward jerking nystagmus correcting a slow upward drift of the eyes, often with the complaint of oscillopsia. It is associated with structural lesions at the cervicomedullary junction and with toxins such as alcohol and anticonvulsants.

5. Upbeat nystagmus—Rapid upward jerking nystagmus correcting a slow downward drift of the eyes. It may occur congenitally, with lesions of the cerebellar vermis or medulla, or after meningitis.

6. Gaze paretic nystagmus—Similar to endpoint nystagmus, except that it occurs in a less extreme position of gaze and is of greater amplitude. It is caused by parietooccipital, cerebellar, and brainstem lesions that affect the conjugate gaze mechanism.

7. Central vestibular nystagmus—Horizontal and rotary jerk nystagmus on lateral gaze, usually jerking to the side opposite the lesion. It is usually not associated with vertigo, tinnitus, or deafness; it may be bidirectional, beating to the right in right gaze and to the left in left gaze, or even vertical on vertical gaze; and it is usually a sign of demyelinating disease, stroke, encephalitis, or tumor.

8. Peripheral vestibular nystagmus—Horizontal and rotary jerk nystagmus on later gaze, opposite the side of the lesion. It is caused by lesions of the labyrinth or eighth cranial nerve.

The most common oscillations in children are as follows:

1. Congenital nystagmus—A conjugate, principally jerk nystagmus that becomes apparent in the perinatal period, often with a null zone, or position with least nystagmus, in a particular gaze position, thus causing anomalous head posture to achieve better vision (Figs. 19-1–19-4).

2. Latent or manifest latent nystagmus—A conjugate, jerk nystagmus evoked or worsened by occlusion of one eye, occurring in patients with strabismus and/or amblyopia. In some patients this type of nystagmus

may be damped, or decreased in intensity, by adducting one eye, creating esotropia.

3. Spasmus nutans—Defined by the symptom triad of anomalous head posture, nystagmus, and head bobbing, typically in children of age 2 and under. It may be rarely associated with chiasmatic glioma or subacute necrotizing encephalomyopathy.

Congenital nystagmus may be associated with a wide variety of nonstrabismic ocular diseases, including

1. Albinism
2. Achromatopsia—A congenital abnormality of the retina with complete loss of color vision, diminished visual acuity to 20/200 to 20/400, photophobia, and nystagmus
3. Aniridia—A congenital absence of all or part of the iris
4. Congenital cataracts
5. Congenital optic nerve disease

If unilateral nystagmus is detected, the following diagnoses should be considered:

1. Spasmus nutans
2. Internuclear ophthalmoplegia
3. Amblyopia
4. Strabismus
5. Blindness
6. Brainstem disease
7. Superior oblique myokymia—An unusual eye movement phenomenon generally considered to be a uniocular rotary microtremor, often treated with carbamazepine

WORKUP

1. History of onset—Anomalous head posture or nystagmus that is acquired past infancy may be a sign of central nervous system lesion. Important neurologic history includes developmental delay, seizures, and meningitis.

2. Neurologic and genetic examination to rule out an obvious cause of nystagmus or anomalous head posture and to help identify any genetic syndrome, such as oculocutaneous albinism.

3. Ophthalmologic examination and referral
   a. Detailed examination to identify any structural abnormality of the eyes or strabismus.
   b. Eye movement recordings may be key in identifying the type of nystagmus (Figs. 19-5–19-8).

c. Electroretinography is used to identify retinal abnormalities.
d. Visual evoked potentials are useful in identifying lesions in the visual pathway.
e. Imaging of the brain is important for ruling out structural central nervous system lesions.
4. Orthopedic referral if all of the above are negative.

TREATMENTS

1. Treatment of any central nervous system lesion
2. Adjustment or discontinuation of medications or drugs causing nystagmus
3. Amblyopia treatment by providing glasses, patching, and/or treating structural anomalies such as cataracts
4. Correction of refractive errors with glasses or contact lenses
5. Surgery, when indicated, to
   a. Correct strabismus
   b. Move the null zone in congenital nystagmus to the primary (straight head) gaze position, by moving the location of extraocular muscle attachments on the globe
   c. Repair ptosis

CONCLUSIONS

Any anomalous head posture or nonphysiologic nystagmus warrants a thorough evaluation. In some cases, the cause may be a life-threatening condition for which early treatment could be of paramount importance.

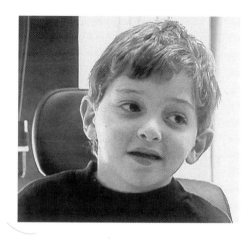

Figure 19-1 *A child with a preferred right face/head turn due to congenital nystagmus with a gaze null (place in space where the nystagmus is least and vision best) to the left.*

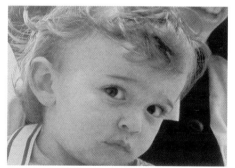

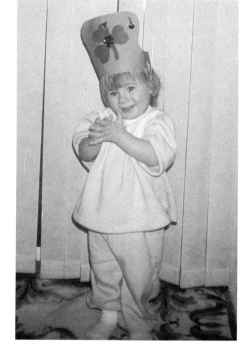

Figures 19-2 and 19-3 *These are children with preferred head tilts due to congenital nystagmus (Fig. 19-2) with a "torsional" null position and strabismus (Fig. 19-3). When they straighten their heads or tilt in the opposite direction shown in the figures, their nystagmus intensity and strabismus increase (decreasing vision and/or causing double vision).*

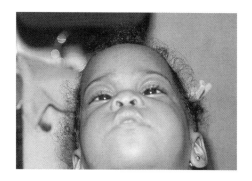

Figure 19-4 *This picture shows a child with a preferred chin-up head posture due to congenital nystagmus with a null position in downgaze.*

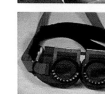
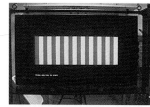
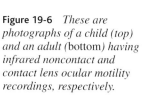
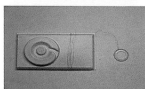

Figure 19-5 *These are photographs of examination chair and stimulus apparatus (top, right, and left), noncontact infrared eye movement recording goggles (bottom left), and contact lens coil (bottom right) used for ocular motility recordings.*

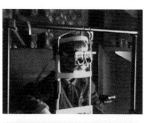
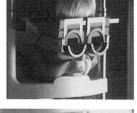
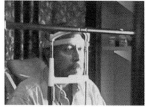
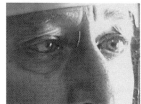

Figure 19-6 *These are photographs of a child (top) and an adult (bottom) having infrared noncontact and contact lens ocular motility recordings, respectively.*

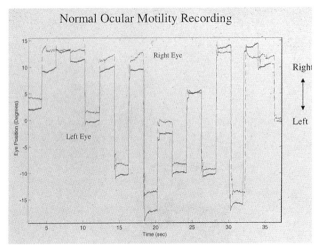

Figure 19-7 *This is an example of an ocular motility recording from a normal patient making rapid back-and-forth eye movements (saccades). There are no involuntary movements.*

Ocular Motility Recording
Congenital Nystagmus

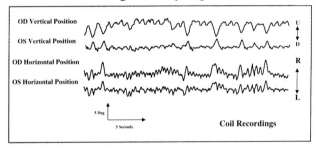

Figure 19-8 *This is an example of a contact lens ocular motility recording of a patient with congenital nystagmus and seesaw nystagmus. The two horizontal tracings on the bottom show the involuntary back-and-forth eye movements. The two vertical tracings on the top show periods of "dysconjugate" movements (e.g., the right eye moves down while the left eye moves up) characteristic of seesaw nystagmus.*

SELECTED REFERENCES

Abadi RV, Pascal E: Periodic alternating nystagmus in humans with albinism. *Invest Ophthalmol Vis Sci* 35:4080–4086, 1984.

Albright AL et al: Spasmus nutans associated with optic gliomas in infants. *J Pediatr* 105:778–785, 1984.

Deskin RW: Sandifer syndrome: a cause of torticollis in infancy. *Int J Pediatr Otorhinolaryngol* 32:183–185, 1995.

Gradstein L et al: Congenital periodic alternating nystagmus: diagnosis and management. *Ophthalmology* 104:918–929, 1997.

Hertle RW, Zhu X: Oculographic and clinical characterization of thirty-seven children with anomalous head postures, nystagmus, and strabismus: the basis of a clinical algorithm. *J Am Assoc Pediatr Ophthalmol Strabismus* 4:25–32, 2000.

Khawam E, el Baba F, Kaba F: Abnormal ocular head postures: parts I, II, III. *Ann Ophthalmol* 19:347–349, 353; 393–395, 399; 428–434; 466–472, 1987.

Kushner BJ: Infantile uniocular blindness with bilateral nystagmus: a syndrome. *Arch Ophthalmol* 113:1298–1300, 1995.

Shallo-Hoffmann J, Faldon M, Tusa RJ: The incidence and waveform characteristics of periodic alternating nystagmus in congenital nystagmus. *Invest Ophthalmol Vis Sci* 40:2546–2553, 1999.

VISION DEVELOPMENT, TESTING, AND VISUAL SCREENING

DAVID B. GRANET

The development of vision and visual responses follows regular milestones. Table 20-1 summarizes clinical aspects of visual development.

VISION SCREENING METHODS

DEFINITION OF TERMS

Routine measurement of vision tests a person's ability to recognize smaller and smaller letters or forms. The angle that the smallest recognizable letter or form subtends on the retina is a measure of visual acuity. Other aspects of vision and visual function that can be measured during an office examination include visual field, color vision, stereopsis (fine depth perception), and contrast sensitivity. Amblyopia and strabismus are significant causes of ocular morbidity and visual disturbances (see Chaps. 7 and 13). Vision screening is the method used to identify these problems or the disorders that are likely to cause them. Amblyopia and strabismus affect 2% to 5% of the population, or a prevalence rate in the United States of roughly 10 million children. This leads to about 100,000 new cases of permanent amblyopia each year. Visual problems in children have a prevalence rate of about 20%. Strabismus also has a large psychosocial impact in children.

Despite evidence that early detection and intervention can decrease the consequences of strabismus and other conditions that lead to amblyopia, studies find that pediatricians are not consistently performing vision screening. Data from the Pediatric Research in Office Settings (PROS network) survey showed that only about one-fourth of primary care physicians test for

binocularity at 3 years of age and about 10% said they test for binocularity among 2-year-olds (26% in both years). In 1993 as in 1988, the majority of pediatricians routinely tested for visual acuity among patients 4 to 6 years of age. However, only one-third of pediatricians reported testing patients for visual acuity at 3 years of age, and very few (6% in 1993 and 5% in 1988) tested patients at 2 years of age. It is true that there are difficulties in performing vision screening in the pediatric population. Infants and younger (preverbal) children are unable to provide subjective responses to visual acuity testing and may not be able to cooperate with testing of ocular alignment or stereo acuity.

Due to the large numbers of children with amblyopia, the National Institutes of Health has made it a priority to improve detection in infants and young children. Vision screening should be performed for a child at the earliest age that is practical, because a small child rarely complains that one eye is not seeing properly.

TECHNIQUES FOR VISION SCREENING IN THE PEDIATRIC POPULATION

1. The Bruckner (Red) Reflex (Fig. 20-1)—
A direct ophthalmoscope is held approximately 18 in from the child and focused. This allows gross evaluation of the red reflex for variation from eye to eye and indicates problems ranging from ocular media opacities (tumors, cataracts, etc.) to refractive errors and ocular misalignment.
2. Corneal (Hirschberg) Reflexes (Fig. 20-2)—
A penlight or muscle light is shone at the

Table 20-1 CLINICAL ASPECTS OF VISUAL DEVELOPMENT

Age	Milestones	Vision	Anatomic Changes
30 weeks' gestational age	Blink to light		Tunica vasculosa regressing
31–32 weeks' gestational age	Pupils react		Risk for retinopathy of prematurity decreasing
Birth	Horizontal gaze in place; intermittent strabismus frequently present	20/400	Anterior-posterior length 17 mm (⅔ of the adult size)
Birth–3 weeks	Early fixation, naso-temporal asymmetry for eye movements	20/200	Most children hyperopic (farsighted)
2 months	Vertical gaze in place; color developing; central, steady gaze; early binocularity		Optic nerve completes myelinization
3–4 months	Good fixing and following, accommodation begins, good alignment		Fovea develops
6 months	Normal ocular alignment	20/40–20/150	Iris pigmentation 90% complete
1 year	Visual field adultlike	20/20–20/60	Infantile esotropia best treated by now
Birth–6 years	Risk for amblyopia greatest	20/20–20/40	Eye growth > 95% complete
6–12 years	Neural plasticity diminishing	20/20	Hyperopia diminishes, myopia appears
12 years	End amblyopic sensitivity		

patient while maintaining his or her attention. This allows evaluation of ocular alignment by observation of the location of the corneal light reflexes.

3. Cover Test (Test for Ocular Alignment and Unequal Vision)—Hold a small interesting toy (that does not make noise) in front of the child (Fig. 20-3). Cover one eye first, then the other (Fig. 20-4). If the child's behavior is different with one eye viewing, then a significant ocular preference may be present. Observation of ocular fixation also allows determination of alignment (strabismus evaluation).

4. Motility Evaluation—An object is moved (with or without sound) to induce a following response of the eyes. This allows evaluation of extraocular movements as well as cranial nerves III, IV, and VI.

5. Preferential Looking Test (Fig. 20-5)—A commercially available form of "forced" preferential looking are the Teller Acuity Cards. These make use of an infant's visual preference for high-contrast black and white stripes over amorphous gray. The child is presented with a series of cards with black-and-white stripes on one side and a matched-luminance gray target on the other side. The tester observes the fixation response of the infant and determines the threshold (increasing spatial frequency [number of black and white stripes]) the child sees.

6. Preliterate Charts (Figs. 20-6 and 20-7)—Charts that do not rely upon knowledge of letters, such as the "tumbling E" or the Allen picture kindergarten test, are likely to overestimate (Allen) or underestimate

("E") vision, depending on the test. These tests are helpful in getting a range of vision in children but may not accurately quantitate vision, making amblyopia diagnosis and treatment difficult.

7. Matching Tests (Fig. 20-8)—These tests of vision do *not* rely on verbal responses of the child. The "HOTV" and Lea tests are two of these types. By removing verbal response from the requirement, younger children can more easily be tested.

8. Letter Charts—Black letters on a white background that subtend known visual angles of resolution at fixed distances are most commonly used in adults and older children. The standard testing method is the Snellen chart (Fig. 20-9), which is over 100 years old. A newer presentation technique, the Early Treatment of Diabetic Retinopathy Study (ETDRS) chart (Fig. 20-10), incorporates a logarithmic score and more letters per line.

9. Stereopsis Test (Fig. 20-11)—Testing of binocularity most commonly utilizes polarized images. Examples include the Titmus and Randot tests. The child indicates which objects appear three-dimensional. These tests determine the brain's ability to perceive "fine" depth perception or stereopsis. This can be used to screen children for strabismus, because even small deviations will have diminished stereopsis.

10. Visual Field Testing—Although visual field testing is not part of routine screening, simple methods such as the "arc perimeter" can be used to test the visual fields of young children (Figs. 20-12 and 20-13).

11. New Approaches—A National Institutes of Health priority calls specifically for the study of better public health methods for testing visual function in preverbal children. The development of photoscreening (Fig. 20-14) has been one major attempt in this direction. In this technique, a photograph enhancing the Bruckner (red) reflex and capturing the corneal reflex is taken.

The photograph is evaluated either by hand (Polaroid photos) or by computer (digital images). Newer chartlike methods have taken advantage of our better understanding of a child's response and utilize contrast sensitivity (Lea symbols).

CURRENT RECOMMENDATIONS FOR VISION SCREENING OF INFANTS AND CHILDREN

1. Neonate and Well-Child Examinations—Perform external (penlight) examination of pupillary response, surface abnormalities of the eye, and surrounding tissues. Test ocular alignment using corneal reflections. Use an ophthalmoscope to view the red reflexes.

2. Preschool Years (up to 5 Years of Age)—Perform external (penlight) examination of pupillary response, surface abnormalities of the eye, and surrounding tissues. Test ocular alignment using corneal reflections or cover test. Use an ophthalmoscope to view the red reflexes. Test monocular visual acuity by picture chart, matching chart, or letters.

3. School-Age Children (Greater than 5 Years of Age)—Assess monocular visual acuity using the Snellen chart. Perform external (penlight) examination of pupillary response, surface abnormalities of the eye, and surrounding tissues. Test ocular alignment using corneal reflections or cover test. Use an ophthalmoscope to view the red reflexes.

CONCLUSIONS

Amblyopia and strabismus can be successfully treated if detected early in their course. Pediatricians are the primary contact point for young children and therefore are the natural source for vision screening. Implementing both available and newer techniques would allow early referral and thus a decrease in morbidity from these significant ocular problems.

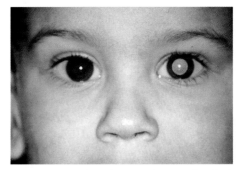

Figure 20-1 *This photograph includes both eyes and has a noticeably diminished red reflex in the patient's right eye. This is consistent with a media opacity (cataract, retinal detachment), strabismus, or a significant refractive error in the eye.*

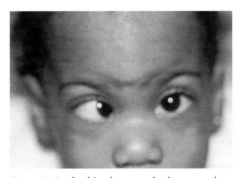

Figure 20-2 *In this photograph, the corneal light reflex is only centered in the left pupil (Hirschberg light reflex), indicating strabismus (in this case esotropia).*

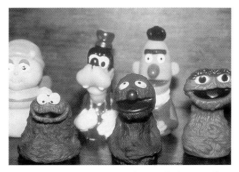

Figure 20-3 *Many types of "toys" that can be used to attract the visual attention of infants to check fixation and following movements of the eyes (normally present by 6 weeks of age).*

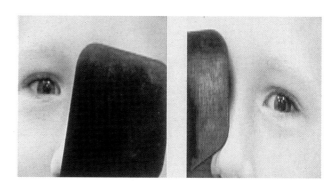

Figure 20-4 *This photograph shows a cover test performed. First the left eye is covered and uncovered, looking for movement of that eye. This is then repeated on the right eye, looking for movement in that eye.*

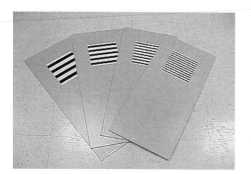

Figure 20-5 *Teller Acuity Cards. The child will preferentially look at the side of the card with the black and white stripes. There is an increasing level of fixation difficulty in the cards presented, as the number of stripes increases on each card.*

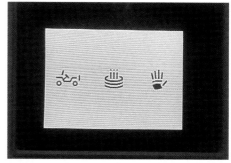

Figure 20-6 *Various "Allen" pictures commonly used to test acuity in preschool children. Although these remain popular, they may be difficult for the contemporary child to recognize and they tend to overestimate visual acuity.*

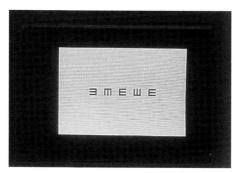

Figure 20-7 *"Tumbling E" optotype test. Although this is a more valid test of vision, the high incidence of left-right or up-down confusion present in the preschool age group makes this test unreliable.*

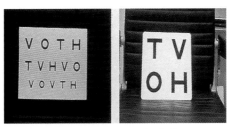

Figure 20-8 *Presentation method of HOTV matching letters (*on the left*) and the "matching" card (*on the right*) that is placed on the child's lap. This test requires no verbal cooperation, making it much more useful in preverbal or nonverbal children.*

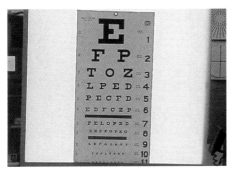

Figure 20-9 *Standard Snellen chart present in many places where vision is measured. The limitations of this test include the facts that only 1 to 3 letters are available for low-vision testing; there is no logarithmic scale of acuity; and it has fixed, common letter presentations.*

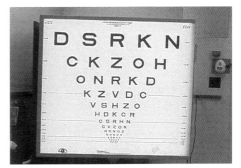

Figure 20-10 *Backlighted Early Treatment of Diabetic Retinopathy Study (ETDRS) chart. This system has numerous changeable letter presentations, records vision in a logarithmic fashion, and includes more letters for low-vision evaluation.*

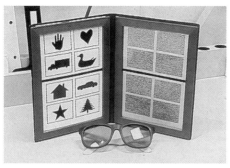

Figure 20-11 *A set of "stereo" plates used for testing stereopsis (fine depth perception) in children. The child wears the polarized glasses and then points to the circle or animal that "jumps" off the page. The use of a combination of monocular visual acuity testing and stereopsis testing is the most sensitive and specific methodology that can be employed by a visual screening program.*

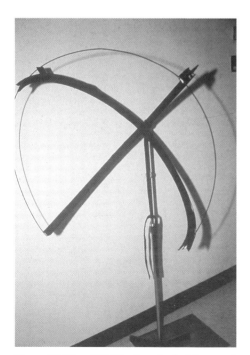 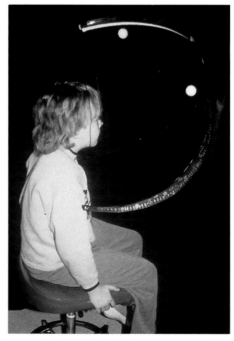

Figures 20-12 and 20-13 *A method of "arc perimetry" designed to test the visual field of toddlers and young children. A white ball travels from the periphery to the center along an arc perimeter (Fig. 20-12) while the child fixes on another ball straight ahead (Fig. 20-13). As soon as the child perceives the peripheral ball, a point on the perimeter is measured, indicating the extent of the visual field in that direction.*

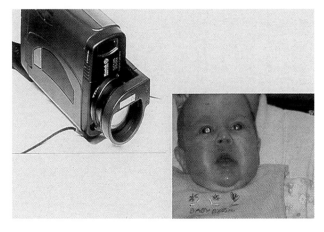

Figure 20-14 *A digital camera especially designed to "capture" the red reflex in both eyes and send that image to a computer. The computer will process the image and help determine if the child needs to be consulted by an eye-care professional. This is one of a number of "photo-screening" devices (left) and the photograph of the "red reflexes" (right) it produces.*

SELECTED REFERENCES

Granet DB et al: A new objective digital computerized vision screening system. *J Pediatr Ophthalmol Strabismus* 36(5):251–256, 1999.

LaRoche GR: Detection, prevention, and rehabilitation of amblyopia. *Curr Opin Ophthalmol* 9(5):10–4, 1998.

Lennerstrand G, Jakobsson P, Kvarnstrom G: Screening for ocular dysfunction in children: approaching a common program. *Acta Ophthalmol Scand* 73(Suppl) 214:26–38; discussion 39–40, 1995.

Limburg H et al: Results of school eye screening of 5.4 million children in India—a five-year follow-up study. Screening for vision problems in pediatric practice. *Acta Ophthalmol Scand* 77(3):310–314, 1999.

Magramm I: Amblyopia: etiology, detection, and treatment. *Pediatr Rev* 13(1):7–14, 1992.

Olitsky SE, Nelson LB: Common ophthalmologic concerns in infants and children. *Pediatr Clin North Am;* 45(4):993–1012, 1998.

Simons BD et al: Pediatric photoscreening for strabismus and refractive errors in a high-risk population. *Ophthalmology* 106:1073–1080, 1999.

REFRACTIVE ERRORS

DAVID F. PLOTSKY

DEFINITION OF TERMS

Clear vision requires a match between the length of an eye and the power of its various refracting surfaces (cornea and lens). A mismatch leads to errors of refraction, resulting in decreased vision. The three main types of refractive errors include hyperopia, myopia, and astigmatism. If the power of the refracting surfaces of the eye is too low for its length (a "short" eye), hyperopia exists. If the power of the refracting surfaces of the eye is too high for its length (a "long" eye), this causes myopia. When the refractive power of an eye varies in different "clock hour" meridians, the eye has astigmatism. Refractive errors may exist in the absence of any identifiable ocular pathology and may run in families. Any pathologic process that affects the size *or* shape of any ocular component may cause or exacerbate refractive errors. The *diopter* is the term used to quantitate refractive error. A lens of 1 diopter of refractive power bends light (refracts) a total of 1 cm at a distance of 1 m from the refracting surface of the lens. By convention, convex surfaces (cause light to converge) are considered to have "plus" (+) power and concave surfaces (cause light to diverge) are considered to have "minus" (−) power (Figs. 21-1–21-4).

DETERMINATION OF REFRACTIVE ERROR

In older children and adults, "subjective" refraction using a Phoropter or trial lens set is the gold standard for determining refractive errors. In preverbal or nonverbal children and adults, "objective" refraction methods are used. This can now be accomplished with var-

ious computer-driven automated methods. The use of retinoscopy as an objective refraction method has a long and well-established record. This is the method most often used by eye-care professionals to diagnose and quantitate refractive errors in children. By first eliminating voluntary accommodation, cycloplegic eye drop medication prior to retinoscopy or automated refraction provides the best way of consistently quantitating refractive errors in children. The anticholinergic drop cyclopentolate 1% is most commonly used, often in combination with sympathomimetic drops (Figs. 21-5–21-9).

CLINICAL CONSIDERATIONS

HYPEROPIA

This is the common refractive status of the normal infant; 1 to 2 diopters of hyperopia frequently remain through early childhood. This tends to increase to about age 6, whereupon it diminishes. Relatively large amounts of uncorrected hyperopia (≥4 diopters) may cause asthenopia, headache, fatigue, and reading aversion. Hyperopia of any amount, but usually more than 3–4 diopters, may be associated with esotropia and amblyopia. Eyes with high hyperopia may be small and have shallow anterior chambers, crowded optic discs, and short axial length (Fig. 21-10).

MYOPIA

Myopia is infrequently present at birth. Childhood myopia is most often found at vision screening examinations or while investigating complaints of blurred vision. Decreased distance vision due to myopia is rarely linked to amblyopia. Some systemic diseases such as Marfan's syndrome or Stickler syndrome are associated with very high levels (pathologic) of myopia. Myopia is often seen in children who have had retinopathy of prematurity. Pathologic myopic eyes tend to have long axial lengths (>30 mm; normal eye, 25 mm) and may have scleral crescents, optic disc anomalies, retinal thinning with tears and detachments, and macular abnormalities (Fig. 21-11).

ASTIGMATISM

All optical parts of the eye have slightly toric surfaces (varied curvature; i.e., shaped like the bowl of a teaspoon, not a sphere). When toricity is large due to increased irregular surfaces of the cornea, lens, or retina, astigmatism sufficient to decrease vision exists. A pathologic process affecting the cornea or lens may be found at any age, but significant astigmatism is usually not found in infants. Most types of astigmatism in children are caused by an exaggeration of the normal toricity of the cornea. This exaggeration is due to unknown combinations of genetic, familial, and environmental factors. Upper lid ptosis, chalazia, and capillary hemangiomas of the eyelid may be directly responsible for significant astigmatism. Keratoconus, a developmental disease of the corneal stroma, causes pathologic levels of astigmatism. Astigmatism may be associated with many other forms of ocular pathology, including iris cysts, cataracts, and retinal or choroidal masses (Figs. 21-12 and 21-13).

GENERAL PRESCRIBING GUIDELINES

HYPEROPIA

1. >3 diopters in an older child or if there is any evidence of amblyopia
2. If the child has unexplained decreased vision or associated strabismus
3. ≥1.5 diopters of anisometropia (difference between the eyes in refraction)
4. If the child has low vision, especially with high hyperopia

MYOPIA

1. Any myopia resulting in decreased vision for age or causing distance symptoms
2. >1 diopter in a symptomatic older child with decreased distance vision
3. Anisometropia if amblyopia is present; optional if no decreased vision or symptoms
4. If the child has associated strabismus, especially exotropia

ASTIGMATISM

1. Full correction of astigmatism in a child with decreased vision and/or symptoms
2. Full correction of astigmatism causing amblyopia
3. >2 diopters in nonverbal children
4. Any degree of anisometropic astigmatism if symptoms or amblyopia present
5. >2 diopters of anisometropic astigmatism if no amblyopia or symptoms

OPHTHALMIC DISEASE IN SCHOOL-AGE CHILDREN

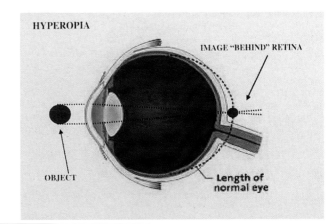

Figure 21-1 *A schematic drawing of a hyperopic eye. Because the overall length of the eye is too short for the refractive power of the cornea and lens, the image is focused behind the retina. This results in an unfocused image presented to the retina and brain.*

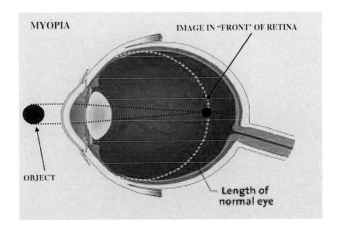

Figure 21-2 *A schematic drawing of a myopic eye. Because the overall length of the eye is too long for the refractive power of the cornea and lens, the image is focused in front of the retina. This results in an unfocused image presented to the retina and brain.*

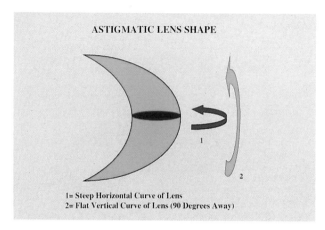

ASTIGMATIC LENS SHAPE

1= Steep Horizontal Curve of Lens
2= Flat Vertical Curve of Lens (90 Degrees Away)

Figure 21-3 *A schematic drawing of an astigmatic lens. The surface of the lens is not uniform in each meridian. The most powerful refractive surface is in the horizontal plane (e.g., 180°), and the least powerful refractive meridian is vertical (e.g., 90°). If the cornea and/or natural lens of the eye have this exaggerated shape, the resulting image is focused in two different meridians, presenting a "sloppy" unfocused image to the brain.*

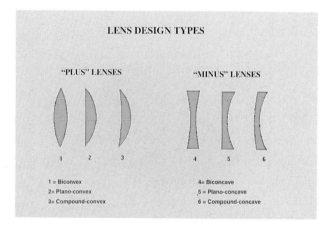

LENS DESIGN TYPES

"PLUS" LENSES

1 = Biconvex
2 = Plano-convex
3 = Compound-convex

"MINUS" LENSES

4 = Biconcave
5 = Plano-concave
6 = Compound-concave

Figure 21-4 *Schematic drawings of the various lens designs. A "plus" lens by convention causes light to converge, whereas a "minus" lens causes light to diverge. Plus lenses are used to treat hyperopia, and minus lenses are used to treat myopia.*

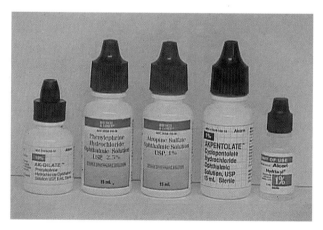

Figure 21-5 *Various eye drops that are used prior to refraction in infants and children. The two classes of drugs used include those that dilate the pupil (mydriatics) and those that paralyze the lens's ability to accommodate (cycloplegics).*

OPHTHALMIC DISEASE IN SCHOOL-AGE CHILDREN

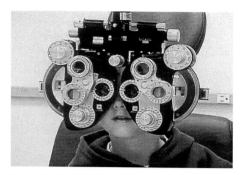

Figure 21-6 *This figure shows a patient undergoing subjective refraction using a Phoropter.*

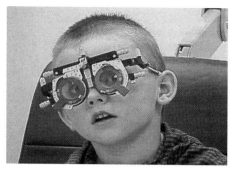

Figure 21-7 *A patient undergoing subjective refraction using trial frames.*

Figure 21-8 *A patient undergoing objective refraction using retinoscopy.*

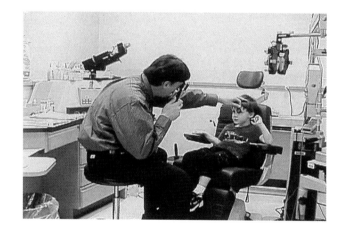

Figure 21-9 *A patient undergoing objective refraction using an automated refraction computer. This method may be inaccurate if the child's eyes are not under the influence of cycloplegia.*

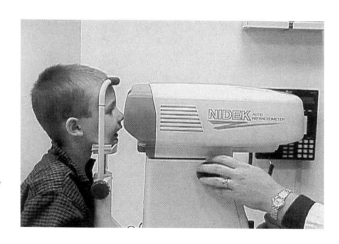

REFRACTIVE ERRORS

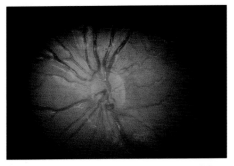

Figure 21-10 *The crowded appearance of the optic nerve of a patient with high hyperopia.*

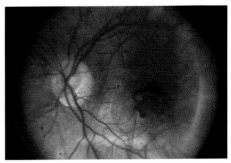

Figure 21-11 *The retinal pathology associated with high myopia. A "scleral crescent" is seen around an optic nerve with a large and displaced optic cup. The macula shows chorioretinal changes consistent with previous damage, e.g., tearing or blood.*

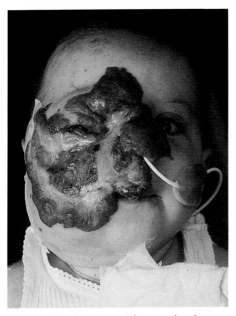

Figure 21-12 *A patient with severe head and facial hemangiomatosis. The massive facial and periocular hemangiomas caused deprivation amblyopia and significant astigmatism of the corneas.*

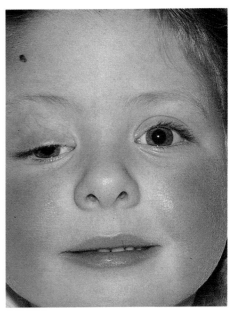

Figure 21-13 *A patient with unilateral congenital ptosis of the upper lid on the right eye. Because the lid has been in this position for 4 years, it has contributed to the development of significant astigmatism in the right eye.*

OPHTHALMIC DISEASE IN SCHOOL-AGE CHILDREN

SELECTED REFERENCES

Bowling EL, Brown MD, Trundle TV: The Stickler syndrome: case reports and literature review. *Optometry* 71(3):177–82, 2000.

Gwiazda J, Thorn F: Development of refraction and strabismus. *Curr Opin Ophthalmol* 9(5):3–9, 1998.

Gwiazda J, Thorn F: Development of refraction and strabismus. *Curr Opin Ophthalmol* 10(5):293–299, 1999.

Harris WF: Astigmatism. *Ophthalmic Physiol Opt* 20(1):11–30, 2000.

Jackson AJ, Saunders KJ: The optometric assessment of the visually impaired infant and young child. *Ophthalmic Physiol Opt* 19(Suppl 2):S49–S62, 1999.

Moore B, Lyons SA, Walline J: A clinical review of hyperopia in young children. The Hyperopic Infants' Study Group, THIS Group. *J Am Optom Assoc* 70(4):215–224, 1999.

Saunders KJ: Early refractive development in humans. *Surv Ophthalmol* 40(3):207–216, 1995.

Spiritus M: Detection, prevention, and rehabilitation of amblyopia. *Curr Opin Ophthalmol* 8(5):11–6, 1997.

ORBITAL TUMORS IN YOUNG CHILDREN

JULIAN D. PERRY and JILL A. FOSTER

LACRIMAL GLAND CYSTS AND TUMORS

DEFINITION OF TERMS

Although lacrimal gland cysts and tumors are uncommon in the pediatric population, both epithelial and lymphoid tumors of the lacrimal gland may arise in young children. Both epithelial and lymphoid tumors of the lacrimal gland present with proptosis and inferonasal displacement of the globe. A palpable mass in the lacrimal gland region may be present. Lymphoid lesions may be bilateral. Imaging studies and rapidity of onset help distinguish between the two types of lesions and guide treatment. Biopsy of a pleomorphic adenoma may result in increased recurrence or malignant degeneration and is contraindicated (Figs. 22-1 and 22-2).

DIFFERENTIAL DIAGNOSIS

1. Benign epithelial cyst
2. Benign mixed tumor (pleomorphic adenoma)
3. Adenoid cystic carcinoma
4. Benign reactive lymphoid hyperplasia
5. Lymphoma
6. Sarcoidosis
7. Dacryoadenitis from viral infection
8. Dermoid cyst
9. Dermolipoma
10. Rhabdomyosarcoma (Fig. 22-3)

WORKUP

1. Determine age of onset and the rate of progression.
2. History and review of systems—Attempt to elicit a history of fever, night sweats, weight loss, or pain and to determine the duration of the symptoms.
3. External examination—Palpate for mass in lacrimal gland region. Is mass adherent to bone in the area of a bony suture? Measure for proptosis (Hertel exophthalmometry) and globe displacement.
4. Complete ocular examination, including evaluation of optic nerve function (visual acuity, color plate testing, visual field examination, presence of an afferent pupillary defect).
5. Computed tomography (CT) is used to evaluate lesions of the lacrimal gland region. Lymphoid lesions tend to mold around the globe. Pleomorphic adenoma tends to indent the globe, and adenoid cystic carcinoma may cause adjacent bony destruction.
6. Incisional biopsy is contraindicated if a pleomorphic adenoma is suspected.

TREATMENTS

1. A rapidly growing lesion (<1 year) causing pain and bony destruction as seen on CT imaging likely represents an adenoid cystic lesion, and incisional biopsy is indicated. If biopsy confirms the diagnosis of adenoid cystic carcinoma, radical surgery (exenteration) and/or chemotherapy and radiotherapy may be considered.
2. A slowly growing (>1 year), painless lesion with evidence of molding on CT may be lymphoma or a pleomorphic adenoma. The lymphoma will have a more homogeneous pattern on the CT scan. If pleomorphic adenoma is not suspected, biopsy may be performed through a lateral approach. If lymphoma is found, systemic workup and oncologic consultation are required. Isolated

lymphoid lesions of the orbit may be treated with radiotherapy. Systemic disease is treated with chemotherapy.

3. A slowly growing (>1 year) lesion with indentation of the globe, significant inferonasal globe displacement, and heterogeneity as seen on CT imaging suggests pleomorphic adenoma. This pathology is unusual in children. En bloc excision with a margin of normal-appearing tissue is indicated.

4. Benign cystic masses in the lacrimal gland may be surgically removed.

CONCLUSIONS

Although unusual in young children, lacrimal gland tumors represent a diagnostic challenge. A thorough history and appropriate imaging studies direct management.

LYMPHANGIOMA

DEFINITION OF TERMS

Lymphangioma is a benign, slowly progressive tumor that is probably congenital but may not become clinically apparent until months or years after birth. Lymphangiomas have been defined as abortive, nonfunctional vascular systems that arborize through variable portions of the orbit. Although they are hemodynamically isolated from the systemic circulation, nutrient vessels within their flimsy walls may be the source of hemorrhage into their lumens. This may transform microscopic channels and cysts into blood-filled "chocolate" cysts. Infections of the upper respiratory tract can cause hyperplasia of the lymphoid tissue with a resultant increase in tissue swelling and proptosis (Figs. 22-5–22-6).

The term *lymphangioma* does not ideally describe these lesions. These lesions are malformations, not autonomous neoplasms, and their anomalous morphogenesis does not produce true lymphatic channels. Recently, orbital vascular malformations have been classified according to their hemodynamic relationships as no-flow, venous-flow, and arterial-flow lesions. Lymphangiomas occupy the no-flow area of this spectrum of orbital vascular malformations. With the advent of good magnetic resonance imaging (MRI) studies, no-flow orbital vascular lesions are being diagnosed more frequently. Typically the clinical onset is in the first few years of life. In many instances, however, it is not recognized until the second decade of life, when the patient presents with abrupt proptosis and periocular soft tissue swelling from spontaneous or traumatic hemorrhage of the lymphangioma. Many patients have lymphangiomas elsewhere, particularly of the palate (Fig. 22-4).

Histopathologically, lymphangioma is an unencapsulated tumor that may diffusely infiltrate the soft tissues of the orbit and the ocular adnexa. The lymphatic channels vary markedly in caliber, ranging from capillary to cavernous. Clear lymph or blood may be present within the lumina of the channels, which are lined by an attenuated endothelium and have a thin wall. The wall around the chocolate cyst is typically more fibrotic.

DIFFERENTIAL DIAGNOSIS

1. Capillary hemangioma
2. Orbital varix
3. Other vascular lesions
4. Schwannoma
5. Neurofibroma (Figure 22-7)
6. Glioma (Figure 22-8)

WORKUP

1. Determine age of onset and the rate of progression.
2. History and review of systems—Abrupt proptosis, sometimes after mild orbital trauma. Increasing proptosis during upper respiratory infection. Increasing proptosis with Valsalva maneuver more likely indicates an orbital varix (venous flow lesion).
3. External examination—Visually inspect the periocular region for an elevated bluish lesion. Determine whether the lesion causes ptosis that crosses the visual axis or indents the globe. Examine the palate for lymphangiomatous lesions. Measure for proptosis (Hertel exophthalmometry) and globe displacement. Examine for signs of exposure keratopathy.
4. Complete ocular examination, including evaluation for amblyopia.
5. There is significant overlap with venous-flow lesions, sometimes termed varices. CT and MRI studies are consistent with the lack of flow and show no evidence of venous or arterial flow. MRI studies may reveal fluid levels within a lymphangioma.

6. Ultrasonography reveals no expansion with increased venous pressure and no venous or arterial flow with Doppler studies.

TREATMENTS

1. If the visual acuity is not threatened in a young child, a period of observation may be indicated.
2. Large hemorrhagic cysts may be aspirated transcutaneously or transconjunctivally to provide temporary relief.
3. Massive tumor and hemorrhage resulting in unacceptable proptosis or compressive optic neuropathy may be treated with surgical debulking. Complications include hemorrhage.
4. Although surgical debulking may result in improvement, continued growth resulting in recurrent proptosis is not uncommon.

CONCLUSIONS

Orbital lymphangiomas represent a slowly progressive hemartomatous no-flow lesion that may cause significant orbital and visual morbidity. The long-term prognosis for acceptable cosmesis and vision is relatively poor.

TERATOMA

DEFINITION OF TERMS

Orbital teratomas arise from congenitally misdirected germ cells. This lesion typically produces massive axial proptosis and associated signs of exposure keratopathy and chemosis. Grossly, the tumors are composed of a mixture of solid and cystic areas. Orbital teratomas are usually benign, and growth is due to an accumulation of secretions within the cystic spaces. Malignant transformation is extremely rare. Benign teratomas do not infiltrate the orbital tissues, and the globe is usually not affected. Histopathologically, teratoma may contain dermal elements, mesenchymal elements, and endodermal tissue.

DIFFERENTIAL DIAGNOSIS

1. Dermoid cyst
2. Lymphangioma
3. Cavernous hemangioma

WORKUP

1. Determine age of onset and the rate of progression.
2. External examination—Look for chemosis and signs of ocular exposure. Measure for proptosis (Hertel exophthalmometry) and globe displacement.
3. Complete ocular examination.
4. CT or MRI studies help define the extent of disease. Teratomas may extend into the temporal fossa and cranial cavity.

TREATMENTS

1. Only after ascertaining the extent of disease can well-planned surgical removal occur.
2. Because the globe is usually not affected, it may be possible in some cases to excise the tumor and retain the eye.
3. A multidisciplinary approach may be needed.

CONCLUSIONS

Teratoma is a rare and usually benign tumor derived from all three germinal layers within the orbit. Surgical excision is the treatment of choice.

MENINGOENCEPHALOCELE

DEFINITION OF TERMS

Meningoencephalocele of the orbit may be divided into anterior and posterior types, depending on where within the orbital bones the defect allows protrusion of the meningeal or brain tissue into the orbit. Anterior meningoencephaloceles are due to bony defects in the area of the ethmoid sinus. These characteristically produce a smooth subcutaneous fluctuant mass on the side of the nose in the region of the medial canthus. Anterior meningoencephaloceles may be bilateral. The posterior type is caused by bony defects in the area of the sphenoid sinus. This produces herniation of brain tissue into the orbit through the superior orbital fissure or the optic foramen. The posterior type may result in pulsating proptosis. In some cases, the brain tissue may lose its connection to the cranial cavity. This results in ectopic brain tissue within the orbit. Meningoencephalocele is associated with other ocular abnormalities, including coloboma, cryptophthalmia, anophthalmia, and microphthalmia (Fig. 22-9).

DIFFERENTIAL DIAGNOSIS

1. Amniotocele
2. Dermoid cyst
3. Mucocele

WORKUP

1. Determine age of onset and the rate of progression.
2. External examination—Visually inspect the periocular region for evidence of colobomas or ocular dysgenesis. Palpate the lesion for fluctuance. Measure for proptosis (Hertel exophthalmometry) and globe displacement.
3. Complete ocular examination.
4. CT or MRI studies help determine the extent of the meningoencephalocele and its relationship to the sinuses, cranial fossa, and brain. Intrathecal contrast may be given to track the connections between the cerebrospinal fluid and the suspected meningoencephalocele.

TREATMENTS

1. Surgical excision is the mainstay of treatment.
2. Surgical management frequently requires a multidisciplinary approach.

CONCLUSIONS

Meningoencephalocele encompasses a spectrum of conditions that result in the prolapse of brain or meningeal tissues through the orbital bones into the orbit. Surgical management depends upon the extent of the lesion.

MUCOCELE

DEFINITION OF TERMS

Mucocele is cystic mass lined with mucous membrane. The lesion begins within a paranasal sinus and may erode into the orbit. Continued expansion into the orbit produces proptosis, orbital congestion, and extraocular motility dysfunction. Orbital signs may be the initial manifestation of the lesion. When a mucocele becomes secondarily infected it is called a *mucopyocele*. Mucoceles that affect the orbit typically arise from the frontal or ethmoid sinuses. Sinus draining outflow obstruction contributes to the formation of a mucocele. Histopathologically, the cyst lining contains sinus respiratory epithelium and an inflammatory reaction within the adjacent tissues. The cyst contains mucus and debris.

DIFFERENTIAL DIAGNOSIS

1. Lacrimal sac mucocele
2. Dermoid cyst
3. Encephalocele

WORKUP

1. Determine age of onset and the rate of progression.
2. History and review of systems—Chronic sinusitis, recurrent upper respiratory infections, failure to thrive.
3. External examination—Palpate the periocular region for a fluctuant superonasal lesion. Measure for proptosis (Hertel exophthalmometry) and globe displacement.
4. Complete ocular examination.
5. Consider workup for cystic fibrosis.
6. CT or MRI studies demonstrate opacification of the sinuses and a cystic mass eroding through the orbital bones into the orbital cavity.

TREATMENTS

1. Surgical excision must remove the entire cyst lining and provide for drainage of the lesion. Sinus drainage must also be reestablished.

CONCLUSIONS

Mucocele is a cystic lesion of the paranasal sinuses eroding into the orbit and producing orbital signs. Surgery is directed at excising the mucocele and providing adequate drainage.

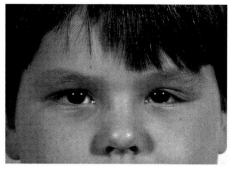
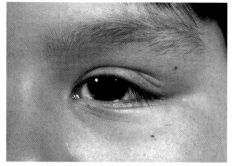

Figures 22-1 and 22-2 *These photographs demonstrate fullness in the left superior temporal orbit with medial displacement of the globe. A close view of the left periocular region in Fig. 22-2 shows the S-shaped distortion of the upper eyelid, which is indicative of a lacrimal gland tumor.*

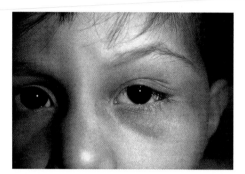

Figure 22-3 *Proptosis and swelling due to an orbital rhabdomyosarcoma.*

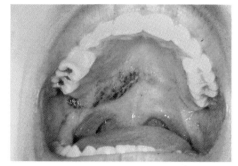

Figure 22-4 *This photograph shows a lymphangioma on the roof of the mouth. The presence of this lesion in a child with proptosis can be a clue to the nature of the orbital process.*

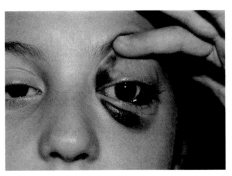

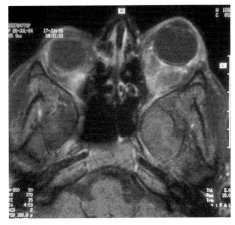

Figures 22-5 and 22-6 *A second clinical feature of lymphangioma, acute hemorrhage. The blood from the orbital hemorrhage has tracked anteriorly into the eyelids and the subconjunctival space. Figure 22-6 is a MRI scan demonstrating the orbital lymphangioma and acute blood collection in this patient.*

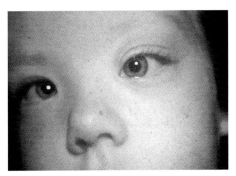

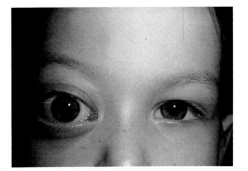

Figures 22-7 and 22-8 *Proptosis of the left eye caused by a neurofibroma (Fig. 22-7) and right eye caused by a glioma (Fig. 22-8).*

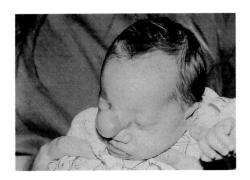

Figure 22-9 *A midline encephalocele involving the right orbit. Encephaloceles result from the herniation of meningeal and brain tissue. These are typically soft and fluctuant on palpation.*

SELECTED REFERENCES

Harris GJ: Orbital vascular malformations: a consensus statement on terminology and its clinical implications. Orbital Society. *Am J Ophthalmol* 127(4):453–455, 1999.

Jakobiec FA, Bonanno PA, Sigelman J: Conjunctival adnexal cysts and dermoids. *Arch Ophthalmol* 96:1040–1049, 1978.

Rootman J et al: Orbital-adnexal lymphangiomas: a spectrum of hemodynamically isolated vascular hamartomas. *Ophthalmology* 93:1558–1570, 1986.

Weiss AH et al: Primary and secondary orbital teratomas. *J Pediatr Ophthalmol Strabismus* 26:44–49, 1989.

PART V

OTHER COMMON CHILDHOOD EYE PROBLEMS

ACCIDENTAL TRAUMA

GORDON BYRNES

DEFINITION OF TERMS

Accidental ocular injuries are a frequent source of childhood emergency room visits. Boys are four times more likely than girls to suffer eye injuries requiring treatment. Roughly 35% of these injuries result in permanent visual impairment and occur with the following frequency: ocular contusions, 51%; penetrating laceration, 28%; nonpenetrating laceration, 16%; foreign bodies and burns, 5%. A majority of ocular injuries occur at home with the child at play, followed in frequency by organized sports, assaults, and motor vehicle accidents. Table 23-1 lists common ocular injuries and the action to be taken.

DIFFERENTIAL DIAGNOSIS (TRAUMA TYPE)

CORNEAL ABRASION AND SUPERFICIAL FOREIGN BODIES

Both corneal abrasion and retained superficial foreign body are common injuries that may cause considerable discomfort, lacrimation, and photophobia. Epithelial abrasion is readily identified with fluorescein staining of the injured tissue. Most epithelial abrasions heal within 24 h if the eye is treated with antibiotic ointment and a pressure patch. Patients that wear contact lenses are at increased risk for corneal ulcer and should not be patched. In cases where foreign body injury potential exists, the eyelids of the injured eye must be everted and inspected to exclude retained matter on the inner eyelid surface (Figs. 23-1–23-5).

Superficial foreign body injury of the cornea or conjunctiva can be detected by careful visual inspection with magnification or a slit lamp. In a cooperative patient, most superficial particles can be removed in the office by irrigating or gently removing the particle. Iron-containing fragments frequently produce a "rust ring" in the surrounding corneal tissue that may be removed by the ophthalmologist if it is located in the visual axis. Once the foreign object is dislodged, the injury is treated as a superficial abrasion.

SHARP LACERATIONS

Eyelid and globe lacerations are most commonly encountered in the setting of multiple traumas involving the face, such as may occur with automobile accident, dog bite injury, or assault. Lacerations involving the eyelids frequently disrupt the specialized array of muscles, tendons, and canaliculi responsible for normal blinking and ocular wetting. Not uncommonly, debris contaminates the wound and poses an additional risk for infection. The evaluation of any eyelid laceration requires both a thorough inspection of the globe and exploration of the wound. A globe laceration is repaired first, creating a watertight seal of the eye. Subsequently, repairing the eyelid laceration must be accomplished in layers, including the reattachment of lacerated muscles, stenting of severed canaliculi, and precise reapproximation of eyelid margins. Imprecise initial closure of the globe or eyelid often results in permanent visual deficit (Figs. 23-6–23-9).

BLUNT INJURY

During blunt ocular trauma, the eye is compressed and deformed as it is retropulsed posteriorly into the orbital fat. In some instances, the compression of orbital tissue leads to orbital floor fracture with entrapment of the inferior rectus muscle, injury to the infraorbital nerve, and opacification of the maxillary sinus with blood. Patients sustaining this injury will note diplopia on attempted upgaze and variable anesthesia in the infraorbital region. Oral antibiotics are commonly prescribed pending surgical repair of the orbital fracture.

Anterior segment deformation during blunt injury may lead to hyphema, iris sphincter tear, cataract, lens subluxation, or ocular rupture. Hyphema has the potential for serious visual consequences from corneal blood staining, glaucoma, or rebleeding. Amblyopia threatens the sight of any young child with media opacification. Aggressive surgical management is often warranted to restore the visual clarity and ocular integrity. Frank rupture through the anterior segment of the eye usually occurs along the limbus and is manifest by a shallow anterior chamber, pupil deformity, hypotony, and hyphema.

Sight-threatening consequences of blunt injury in the posterior segment of the eye include concussive and ocular deformity effects. Disruption of the rod and cone outer segments through transmitted concussive force is manifest as regional retinal whitening (com-motio retinae) and may result in macular hole formation. Full-thickness retinal necrosis may arise near the impact site of the injury and results in permanent loss of retinal tissue. Traumatic retinal dialysis occurs when the ocular deformity exceeds the elasticity of the vitreous base, resulting in tearing of the peripheral retina near the ora serrata. Ocular compression against the optic nerve results in ringlike rupture of the choroid and is associated with subretinal hemorrhage.

Blunt posterior segment globe rupture may have variable signs of presentation that include poor vision, vitreous hemorrhage, reduced ocular motility, hemorrhagic chemosis, deep anterior chamber, reduced intraocular tension, and excessive lacrimation. Eyes suspected of possible rupture require prompt surgical exploration and repair (Figs. 23-10–23-15).

PENETRATING TRAUMA

Ocular penetrating injuries in children typically result from projectiles emitted from a metal-on-metal strike, BB gun or pellet rifle, secondary missiles associated with explosion, or dartlike

---

Table 23-1 ACCIDENTAL OCULAR TRAUMA AND RECOMMENDED ACTIONS

Injury	Action
Blowout fracture	Comprehensive globe evaluation, orbital CT, oral antibiotic coverage; refrain from nose blowing; refer to ophthalmology.
Corneal abrasion	Rule out retained foreign material (evert eyelid); administer antibiotic ointment and cycloplegic; pressure patch for 24 h; recheck. Refer nonhealing abrasion to ophthalmology.
Eyelid laceration	Careful globe evaluation; prompt exploration and repair of laceration by ophthalmology.
Hyphema	Fox shield; cycloplegia; avoid aspirin and reading; prompt ophthalmology referral.
Ocular contusion	Careful globe evaluation; refer to ophthalmology for dilated fundus exam.
Spontaneous subconjunctival hemorrhage	Rule out bleeding diathesis or penetrating injury. Uncomplicated subconjunctival hemorrhage requires no treatment.
Superficial corneal foreign body	Irrigation or mechanical foreign body removal, then treat as corneal abrasion. Refer penetrating foreign body promptly to ophthalmology, protect eye with Fox shield.
Suspected globe rupture	Careful globe evaluation; start IV antibiotic coverage; Fox shield; prompt referral to ophthalmology for exploration and repair.

OTHER COMMON CHILDHOOD EYE PROBLEMS

projectiles. The particle shape, density, and velocity determine the depth of penetration and degree of tissue disruption. Metal-on-metal strikes commonly produce minute, sterile, high-velocity particles that penetrate the eye with minimal signs of overt damage. BBs typically cause marked deformation of the globe before penetration and are associated with a discouraging visual prognosis. Projectiles associated with explosion may include glass, metal, rock, or organic matter, and often pose an increased risk of wound contamination and infection. When media opacity prevents fundus examination, computed tomography (CT) is invaluable in detecting and localizing most intraocular particles. Foreign objects retained within the globe typically require surgical removal, whereas nonorganic particles located within the adnexa can usually be observed (Figs. 23-16–23-18).

BIRTH TRAUMA

During vaginal delivery the eyes and eyelids are at risk for minor traumas and eyelid edema as a result of protracted facial compression. Corneal abrasion is more common with forceps delivery and is usually self-limited. In 11% to 30% of uncomplicated deliveries, fundus examination demonstrates scattered blot or white-centered retinal hemorrhages. The hemorrhages usually are scattered throughout the fundus, clear spontaneously over a few days to a week, and are rarely of visual concern. Serious ocular injuries associated with forceps use include hyphema, corneal edema, lens subluxation, and eyelid ptosis. Aside from the immediate gravity of the injury, any protracted disturbance of the visual axis may result in dense amblyopia (Figs. 23-19–23-21).

WORKUP

1. Full history, allergies, tetanus immunization status
2. Test of vision (Snellen chart, finger counting, hand motions, light perception)
3. Examine for associated head, facial, neck, or systemic injury
4. Protect injured eye with a shield and refer to ophthalmologist

MANAGEMENT OF OCULAR TRAUMA

The evaluation of a child presenting with ocular trauma may be problematic due to an often-incomplete history of the injury as well as difficult patient examination. Any child suspected to harbor a potentially serious ocular injury requires a thorough examination by a trained specialist and may require examination under anesthesia to accomplish the evaluation. When a serious injury is identified or suspected, a Fox shield should be applied to protect the eye, and the child's activity should be minimized as much as practical. Topical antibiotics should be avoided until globe rupture can be excluded, because many drugs are toxic to exposed retinal tissue. Intravenous antibiotics are frequently administered when globe rupture or substantial wound contamination is suspected. An eye considered to harbor a rupture must undergo prompt exploration and repair. A CT scan of the orbit is often performed preoperatively to exclude a foreign body associated with the globe injury. In general, an ophthalmologist should perform the specialized ocular exploration and repair (Fig. 23-22).

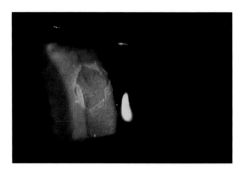

Figure 23-1

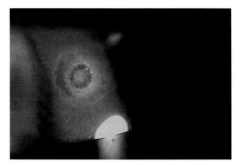

Figure 23-2

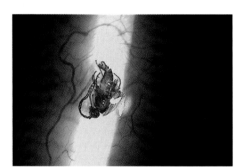

Figure 23-3

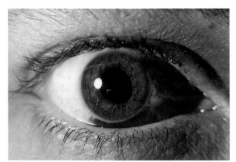

Figure 23-4

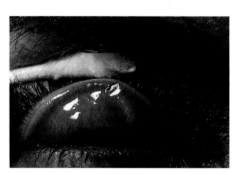

Figure 23-5

Figures 23-1 to 23-5   *Figure 23-1 shows a superficial corneal epithelial abrasion. Figure 23-2 shows a corneal rust ring following removal of an iron-containing foreign body. Figure 23-3 shows an adherent insect on conjunctival epithelium. Figure 23-4 shows a spontaneous subconjunctival hemorrhage, and Fig. 23-5 shows an everted upper eyelid revealing a small metallic foreign body embedded in the tarsus.*

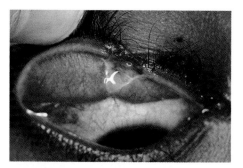

Figure 23-6

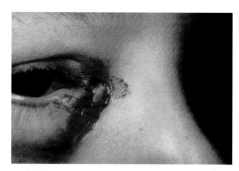

Figure 23-7

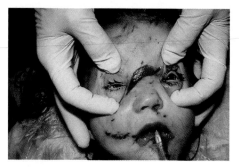

Figure 23-8

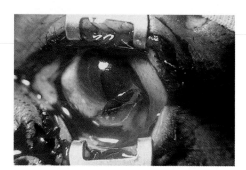

Figure 23-9

Figures 23-6 to 23-9 *Figure 23-6 shows an everted upper eyelid with a full-thickness laceration through the eyelid margin. Figure 23-7 shows a shelved laceration of the lower eyelid extending through the inferior canaliculus medially. Figure 23-8 shows a complex of facial lacerations and punctures following a mauling injury by a large dog. Figure 23-9 shows a combined globe and eyelid laceration. Note the protruding iris tissue within the limbal wound, resulting in a distorted pupil.*

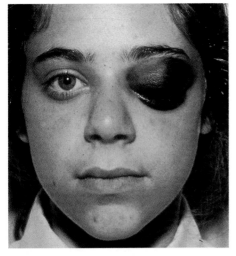

Figure 23-10

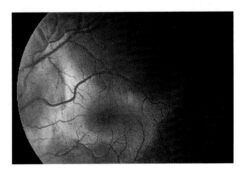

Figure 23-11

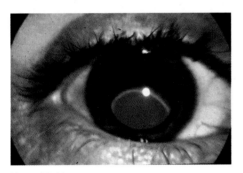

Figure 23-12

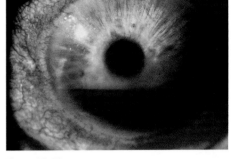

Figure 23-13

OTHER COMMON CHILDHOOD EYE PROBLEMS

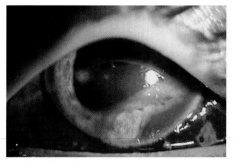

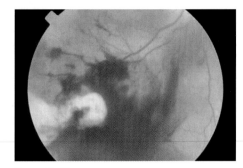

Figure 23-14   **Figure 23-15**

Figures 23-10 to 23-15 *Figure 23-10 shows upper and lower eyelid ecchymosis following blunt trauma. Figure 23-11 shows an anterior segment photograph of a posttraumatic layered hyphema with associated conjunctival injection. Figure 23-12 shows a posttraumatic lens subluxation visible within the red light reflex. Figure 23-13 depicts commotio retinae, which is a whitening of the outer retina following blunt contusion injury. Histopathology of this condition reveals a shearing of the outer segments of the rods and cones. Figure 23-14 shows iris dialysis and subconjunctival hemorrhage following blunt ocular contusion with a paintball projectile. Figure 23-15 shows a fundus photograph demonstrating full-thickness retinal necrosis and retinal hemorrhage corresponding to the paintball impact site.*

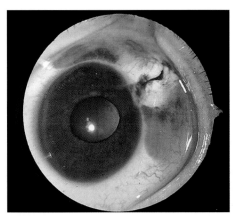

Figure 23-16

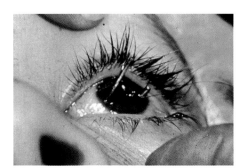

Figure 23-17

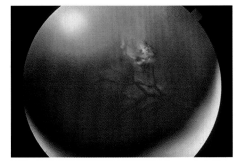

Figure 23-18

Figures 23-16 to 23-18   *Figure 23-16 shows the entrance site of a penetrating injury associated with subconjunctival hemorrhage. The dark material within the scleral wound represents the choroid. Figure 23-17 shows a wire staple penetrating the anterior segment and extending through the cornea. Figure 23-18 shows a small metallic projectile embedded in the surface of the retina. The view is partially obscured by vitreous hemorrhage.*

OTHER COMMON CHILDHOOD EYE PROBLEMS

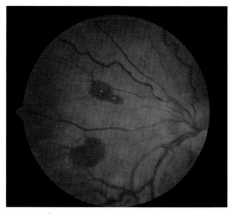

Figure 23-19

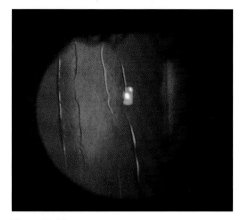

Figure 23-20

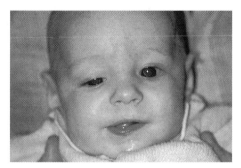

Figure 23-21

Figures 23-19 to 23-21 *Figure 23-19 shows a fundus photograph of blot and white-centered hemorrhages following an uncomplicated vaginal delivery. Figure 23-20 shows the corneal stria visible on retroillumination representing disruptions in Descemet's membrane as a result of corneal compression during forceps delivery. Figure 23-21 shows ptosis of the right upper eyelid following forceps delivery.*

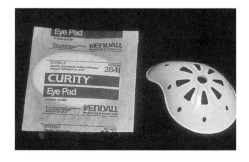

Figure 23-22 *Figure 23-22 shows the gauze eye pad and Fox shield used in patching and protecting the injured eye.*

SELECTED REFERENCES

Cassen JH: Ocular trauma. *Hawaii Med J* 56(10):292–294, 1997.

Coats DK et al: Outpatient management of traumatic hyphemas in children. *Binocul Vision Strabismus Quarterly;* 15(2):169–174, 2000.

Goldberg SH: Ocular and orbital trauma: preventive medicine in ophthalmology. *Curr Opin Ophthalmol* 9(5):39–40, 1998.

Juang PS, Rosen P: Ocular examination techniques for the emergency department. *J Emerg Med* 15(6):793–810, 1997.

Kitchens JW, Danis RP: Increasing paintball related eye trauma reported to a state eye injury registry. *Injury Prevention* 5(4):301–2, 1999.

Negrel AD, Thylefors B: The global impact of eye injuries. *Ophthalmic Epidemiol* 5(3): 143–169, 1998.

Pieramici DJ et al: Open-globe injury. Update on types of injuries and visual results. *Ophthalmology* 103(11):1798–1803, 1996.

CHAPTER 24

SPECTACLES IN INFANTS AND CHILDREN

JOHN ORT

DEFINITIONS OF TERMS

The use of spectacles for the correction of refractive errors in infants and children is one of the most important steps in assuring proper development of the visual system. Providing equally clear images to the retina of a child during development assures that central visual development can proceed. Often the first step in treatment of amblyopia and strabismus involves the use of spectacles. The infant and child require special attention regarding spectacle lens type and frame design. The small pupillary distance and undeveloped nasal bridge require specially designed frames. The use of glass lenses has largely been abandoned in place of "plastic." Children may also require complicated spectacle correction, such as bifocals and aphakic (after cataract surgery) prescriptions. The anatomy of the spectacle includes the material (metal or plastic), temples, hinges, bridge, and "eye wire" (full rim, half-rim, or rimless). Important dimensions include the eye size, bridge size, and temple length. In general, the larger the eye size, the more exaggerated the lens problems, e.g., thickness, weight, and optical aberrations. Using high-index plastic lenses can now reduce these lens problems.

DIFFERENTIAL DIAGNOSIS REQUIRING SPECTACLES

1. Myopia
2. Hyperopia
3. Astigmatism
4. Anisometropia (intereye refractive error differences)
5. Amblyopia
6. Strabismus
7. Aphakia (no lens in the eye)
8. Retinal disease with photophobia
9. Monocular blindness (protection of the only eye)

WORKUP

1. History of material allergies
2. Desired purpose of spectacles (e.g., routine, sports, protection, strabismus correction)
3. Pupillary distance measurements, distant and near vision
4. Temple length measurements

TREATMENTS

1. Appropriate eye size for child and prescription (Figs. 24-1 and 24-2).
2. Frame material—Plastic frames provide molded, "flat" bridges generally necessary in infants. Metal frames come with adjustable nose pads that allow a custom fit on the nose. The newer "memory" metal is lightweight and resists bending and breaking. This frame style may be ideal for active children.
3. Correct bridge and temple fit (Figs. 24-3–24-6).
4. Lens materials—Almost always plastic or polycarbonate (bulletproof). High-index materials are plastic lenses useful for treating large refractive errors in that they minimize lens weight and thickness.
5. Lens style (single vision versus bifocal)—Flat-top (or D) bifocals are preferred and are first fit at the middle of the child's pupil to ensure their use (Figs. 24-7–24-12).

6. Lens color—Both glass and plastic lenses come in a variety of hues and densities. Due to recent knowledge about long-term sun exposure and eye damage, children should have the same opportunity as adults to routinely wear sun protection. Children with photophobia from ocular diseases almost always benefit from tinted lenses.

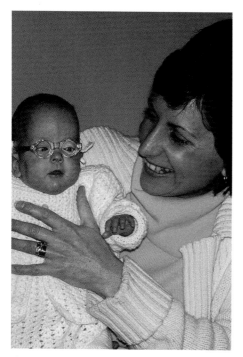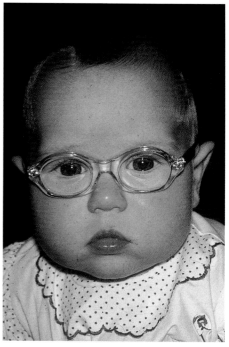

Figures 24-1 and 24-2 *Two infants with well-fitting plastic frames. The child in Fig. 24-1 has bilateral high myopia, and the child in Fig. 24-2 has moderate myopia.*

OTHER COMMON CHILDHOOD EYE PROBLEMS

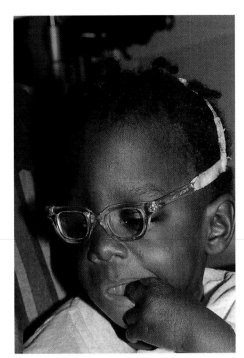

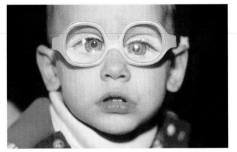

Figures 24-3 and 24-4 *Two toddlers in a style of frame with a flat nasal bridge and temples that are almost all an elastic strap. The child in Fig. 24-3 has high hyperopia due to aphakia, and the child in Fig. 24-4 has myopic astigmatism.*

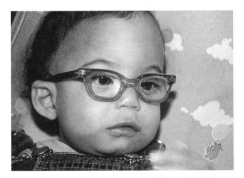

Figure 24-5 *A toddler with unilateral high myopia in the left eye (anisometropia) in a well-fit plastic frame. Notice the appearance of a proper eye size, nasal bridge, and temple length for his age.*

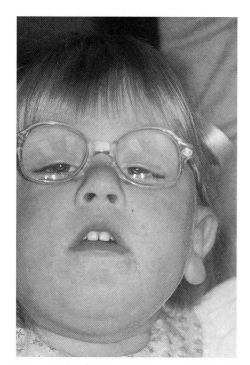

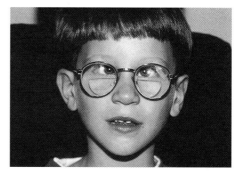

Figures 24-6 and 24-7 *Children fit with bifocal spectacles. In Fig. 24-6 this child is looking through the bifocal to improve her acuity at distance, indicating a need for a change in her distance prescription. Figure 24-7 shows a child with accommodative esotropia in his poorly fit hyperopic glass prescription and flat-top 35-mm bifocals placed too low. This type of bifocal segment is much preferred over the "executive" style bifocal for manufacturing, optical, and cosmetic reasons.*

OTHER COMMON CHILDHOOD EYE PROBLEMS

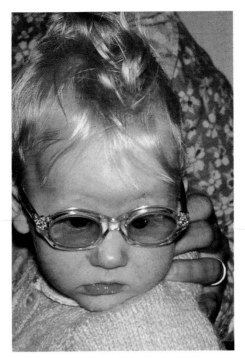

Figure 24-8 *This child with oculocutaneous albinism has amber-tinted lenses in her myopic spectacles to try to decrease her photophobia.*

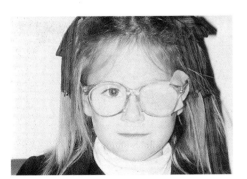 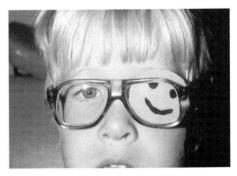

Figures 24-9 and 24-10 *These children are both undergoing occlusion therapy for amblyopia and are using the glasses to help with a patch that does not adhere to the skin. This form of penalization is usually less effective than an adhesive patch, but is better than no occlusion.*

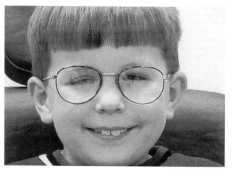 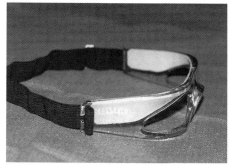

Figures 24-11 and 24-12 *Children need eye protection for many reasons. Figure 24-11 shows a child with monocular blindness due to glaucoma wearing polycarbonate (bulletproof) lenses. Figure 24-12 is one illustration of the many styles of protective spectacles worn during sporting activities.*

SELECTED REFERENCES

Darie H, Crepy P: Sun and skin and eye protection. *Med Trop (Mars)* 57(4):493–496, 1997.

Davis LJ: Complex refractive errors in pediatric patients: cause, management, and criteria for success. *Optom Vis Sci* 75(7): 493–499, 1998.

Hiatt RL: Rehabilitation of children with cataracts. *Trans Am Ophthalmol Soc* 96:473–515; discussion 515–517, 1998.

Hornby SJ et al: Requirements for optical services in children with microphthalmos, coloboma and microcornea in southern India. *Eye* 14(2):219–224, 2000.

Horwood AM: Compliance with first time spectacle wear in children under eight years of age. *Eye* 12(2):173–178, 1998.

Miller JM, Harvey EM: Spectacle prescribing recommendations of AAPOS members. *J Pediatr Ophthalmol Strabismus* 35(1):51–52, 1998.

Pizzarello L et al: A new school-based program to provide eyeglasses: childsight. *J Am Assoc Pediatr Ophthalmol Strabismus* 2(6):372–374, 1998.

Spear TM et al: The effects of strapped spectacles on the fit factors of three manufactured brands of full face piece negative pressure respirators. *Ann Occup Hyg* 43(3):193–199, 1999.

Tishler C, Hertle R: The fitting and dispensing of spectacles to the pediatric patient: a psychological perspective. *Optical Index* 55:25–29, 1980.

OTHER COMMON CHILDHOOD EYE PROBLEMS

INDEX

Note: Page numbers followed by f indicate figures; those followed by t indicate tables.

Retinopathy of prematurity (ROP), 49–54
  classification of, 50, 51f–54f
  Coats' disease versus, 79
  definition of, 49
  differential diagnosis of, 49
  familial exudative vitreoretinopathy versus, 81
  Leber's congenital amaurosis versus, 82
  ocular toxocariasis versus, 80
  persistent hyperplastic primary vitreous versus, 78
  screening for, 50
  treatment of, 50–51, 54f
  workup for, 49–50
  X-linked retinoschisis versus, 83
Retinoschisis, X-linked, 91f
  Coats' disease versus, 79
  familial exudative vitreoretinopathy versus, 81
  Leber's congenital amaurosis versus, 82
  ocular toxocariasis versus, 80
  persistent hyperplastic primary vitreous versus, 78
  Stargardt's disease versus, 83
Retinoscopy, 209f
Retrolental fibroplasia (RLF). See Retinopathy of
    prematurity (ROP)
Rhabdomyosarcomas, orbital, 151–152, 159f, 217f
Rheumatoid arthritis, juvenile, uveitis associated
    with, 183
Rubella, 10t, 12f–13f
Rubeosis iridis, with retinoblastoma, 169f
Rust ring, corneal, 226

Sarcoidosis, 186f
Sclerocornea, 31, 35f
  with Peter's anomaly, 35f
Screening
  for retinopathy of prematurity, 50
  vision, 197–204, 198t
    recommendations for, 199
    techniques for pediatric population, 197–199,
      200f–204f
Seesaw nystagmus, 189–190
Silastic tube placement, for nasolacrimal duct
    obstruction, 115f–116f
Silver nitrate drops, conjunctivitis due to, 7f
Snellen chart, 202f
Spectacles, 233–238
  for accommodative esotropia, 123f
  for amblyopia, 122f
  bifocal, 236f
  indications for, 233
  lenses for, 208f
  protective, 238f
  with tinted lenses, 232, 237f
  treatment using, 233–234, 234f–238f
  workup for, 233
Staphyloma, peripapillary, of optic nerve, 96,
    100f

Stargardt's disease, 83–84, 92f
Stereopsis test, 199, 203f
Steroids, cataracts associated with, 28f
Strabismus, 59–65
  comitant, 120, 123f–124f
  definition of, 59
  diagnosis of, 59–60
  differential diagnosis of, 60, 61f–65f
  noncomitant, 120–121
    in Brown's syndrome, 121, 127f
    in Duane's syndrome, 121, 126f
    with monocular elevation deficiency, 121, 128f
    with superior oblique muscle palsy or
      underaction, 120–121, 125f
  paralytic, in inflammatory myositis, 154f
  with retinoblastoma, 169f
  treatment of, 60–61, 122
  with varicella zoster virus infection, 19f
  workup for, 60, 121–122
Sturge-Weber syndrome, 156f
Styes, 129, 139f
Subconjunctival hemorrhage
  spontaneous, 224t
  traumatic, 108f
    following blunt trauma, 229f
    following penetrating trauma, 230f
Subdural hemorrhage, 109f
Subjective refraction, 209f
Synophthalmia, 42, 46f
Syphilis, 10t, 11f

Telangiectasia, in Coats' disease, 87f
Teller Acuity Cards, 201f
Teratomas, orbital, 215
"Tessier" facial clefts, 72f
Tetraploidy, 70
Thrombophilic disorder, retinopathy of prematurity
    versus, 49
"Tin ear syndrome," 109f
TORCH syndromes, 9–10, 11f, 20f
  treatment of, 9, 10t
Torticollis, 189
Toxocariasis
  macular granulomas in, 89f
  ocular, 80, 89f
Toxoplasmosis
  Aicardi's syndrome versus, 82
  coloboma versus, 79
  congenital, 10t, 14f–15f
  familial exudative vitreoretinopathy versus, 81
  ocular toxocariasis versus, 80
  persistent hyperplastic primary vitreous versus, 78
  recurrent, 134
  Stargardt's disease versus, 83
  X-linked retinoschisis versus, 83
Trauma. See Accidental trauma; Child abuse